The Anatomy of Stretching

Your Illustrated Guide to Flexibility and Injury Rehabilitation

Second Edition

Brad Walker

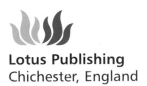

Lotus Publishing
Chichester, England

North Atlantic Books
Berkeley, California

First published in 2007. This revised second edition published in 2011 by
Lotus Publishing
Apple Tree Cottage, Inlands Road, Nutbourne, PO18 8RJ and
North Atlantic Books
P.O. Box 12327
Berkeley, California 94712

Drawings Pascale Pollier and Amanda Williams
Text Design Wendy Craig
Cover Design Jim Wilkie
Printed and Bound by Scotprint

The Anatomy of Stretching is sponsored by the Society for the Study of Native Arts and Sciences, a nonprofit educational corporation whose goals are to develop an educational and cross-cultural perspective linking various scientific, social, and artistic fields; to nurture a holistic view of arts, sciences, humanities, and healing; and to publish and distribute literature on the relationship of mind, body, and nature.

MEDICAL DISCLAIMER: The following information is intended for general information purposes only. Individuals should always see their health care provider before administering any suggestions made in this book. Any application of the material set forth in the following pages is at the reader's discretion and is his or her sole responsibility.

British Library Cataloguing in Publication Data
A CIP record for this book is available from the British Library
ISBN 978 1 905367 29 0 (Lotus Publishing)
ISBN 978 1 55643 596 6 (North Atlantic Books)

The Library of Congress has cataloged the first edition as follows:
Walker, Brad, 1971–
    The anatomy of stretching / Brad Walker.
        p. cm.
    ISBN-13: 978-1-55643-596-6 (pbk.)
    ISBN-10: 1-55643-596-7 (pbk.)
    1. Stretching exercises. I. Title.
    RA781.63.W35 2006
    613.7'182--dc22

                                        2006022377

Contents

How to Use This Book

The Anatomy of Stretching is designed to provide a balance of theoretical information about the fundamentals of stretching and flexibility anatomy and physiology, and the practical application of how to perform 135 unique stretching exercises. All the stretching exercises are indexed according to what part of the body is being stretched and further information is provided on exactly which muscles are being targeted.

As well as a detailed anatomical drawing, each stretch section includes a description of how the stretch is performed, a list of sports and sports injuries that the stretch is most beneficial for, and additional information about any common problems associated with this stretch.

The information about each stretch is presented in a uniform style throughout. An example is given below, with the meaning of headings explained in bold.

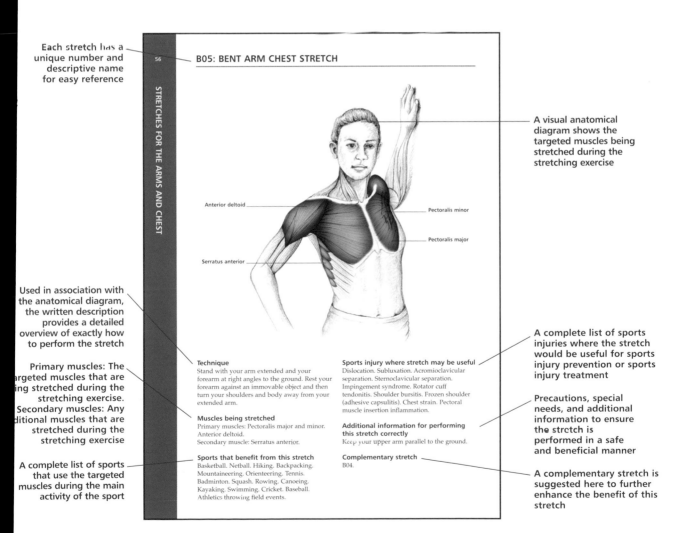

Each stretch has a unique number and descriptive name for easy reference

A visual anatomical diagram shows the targeted muscles being stretched during the stretching exercise

Used in association with the anatomical diagram, the written description provides a detailed overview of exactly how to perform the stretch

Primary muscles: The targeted muscles that are being stretched during the stretching exercise. Secondary muscles: Any additional muscles that are stretched during the stretching exercise

A complete list of sports that use the targeted muscles during the main activity of the sport

A complete list of sports injuries where the stretch would be useful for sports injury prevention or sports injury treatment

Precautions, special needs, and additional information to ensure the stretch is performed in a safe and beneficial manner

A complementary stretch is suggested here to further enhance the benefit of this stretch

---

56 | STRETCHES FOR THE ARMS AND CHEST

B05: BENT ARM CHEST STRETCH

Anterior deltoid
Pectoralis minor
Pectoralis major
Serratus anterior

Technique
Stand with your arm extended and your forearm at right angles to the ground. Rest your forearm against an immovable object and then turn your shoulders and body away from your extended arm.

Muscles being stretched
Primary muscles: Pectoralis major and minor. Anterior deltoid.
Secondary muscle: Serratus anterior.

Sports that benefit from this stretch
Basketball. Netball. Hiking. Backpacking. Mountaineering. Orienteering. Tennis. Badminton. Squash. Rowing. Canoeing. Kayaking. Swimming. Cricket. Baseball. Athletics throwing field events.

Sports injury where stretch may be useful
Dislocation. Subluxation. Acromioclavicular separation. Sternoclavicular separation. Impingement syndrome. Rotator cuff tendonitis. Shoulder bursitis. Frozen shoulder (adhesive capsulitis). Chest strain. Pectoral muscle insertion inflammation.

Additional information for performing this stretch correctly
Keep your upper arm parallel to the ground.

Complementary stretch
B04.

Introduction

The subject of stretching and flexibility has evolved considerably over the last fifteen to twenty years. Long gone are the days when the topic of stretching was relegated to a few pages at the back of books on health and fitness, or when a dozen stick figures performing the most basic of stretching exercises was considered a detailed reference.

Fifteen years ago it was hard to find a text specifically on stretching, but today there are dozens of references. Everything from "New Age" stretching techniques to martial arts stretching and the very detailed clinical application of stretching for academics has been written.

When *The Anatomy of Stretching* was originally published in 2007 it was the first book to cover the topic of anatomy and physiology for stretching and flexibility. Since then others have been written, but no other book on the subject contains more examples of stretching exercises, or is able to take detailed anatomical information and present it in a way that is easy for everyone to understand.

This is where *The Anatomy of Stretching* is different: it is able to take you inside the body and show you both the primary and secondary muscles in action during the stretching process.

The Anatomy of Stretching looks at stretching from every angle, including physiology and flexibility; the benefits of stretching; the different types of stretching; rules for safe stretching; and how to stretch properly. Aimed at fitness enthusiasts of any level, as well as fitness pros, *The Anatomy of Stretching* also focuses on which stretches are useful for the alleviation or rehabilitation of specific sports injuries.

Plus in this second edition, over 20 new stretches have been added; the chapter on physiology has been expanded; more detailed anatomy has been included with each stretching chapter; and a new numbering system has been included to help reference each stretch.

Written as a visual aid for athletes and fitness professionals, *The Anatomy of Stretching* gives readers a balance of theoretical information about the fundamentals of stretching and flexibility anatomy and physiology, and the practical application of how to perform 135 unique stretching exercises.

Divided into stand-alone sections, *The Anatomy of Stretching* does not have to be read from cover-to-cover to take advantage of the information it contains. If you would like to see how a muscle works, refer to Chapter 1; if you would like to know how stretching can help you, have a read through some of the benefits in Chapter 2; and if you would like information on stretches for the hamstrings, look under Chapter 9.

Whether you are a professional athlete or a fitness enthusiast, a sports coach or personal trainer, a physical therapist or sports doctor, *The Anatomy of Stretching* will benefit you.

Brad Walker

1

Flexibility, Anatomy, and Physiology

Fitness and Flexibility

An individual's physical fitness depends on a vast number of components; flexibility is only one of these. Although flexibility is a vital part of physical fitness, it is important to see it as only one spoke in the fitness wheel. Other components include strength, power, speed, endurance, balance, co-ordination, agility, and skill.

Although particular sports require different levels of each fitness component, it is essential to plan a regular exercise or training program that covers all the components of physical fitness. Rugby and American football (gridiron), for example, rely heavily on strength and power; however, the exclusion of skill drills and flexibility training could lead to serious injury and poor performance. Strength and flexibility are of prime concern to a gymnast, but a sound training program would also improve power, speed, and endurance.

The same is true for each individual: while some people seem to be naturally strong or flexible, it would be foolish for such persons to completely ignore the other components of physical fitness. And just because an individual exhibits good flexibility at one joint or muscle group, it does not mean that the entire individual will be flexible. Therefore, flexibility must be viewed as specific to a particular joint or muscle group.

The Dangers and Limitations of Poor Flexibility

Tight, stiff muscles limit our normal range of movement. In some cases, lack of flexibility can be a major contributing factor to muscle and joint pain. In the extreme, lack of flexibility can mean it is difficult, for example, to even bend down or look over our shoulder.

Tight, stiff muscles interfere with proper muscle action. If the muscles cannot contract and relax efficiently, this will result in decreased performance and a lack of muscle movement control. Short, tight muscles also cause a dramatic loss of strength and power during physical activity.

In a very small percentage of cases, muscles that are tight and stiff can even restrict blood circulation. Good blood circulation is vitally important in helping the muscles receive adequate amounts of oxygen and nutrients. Poor circulation can result in increased muscle fatigue and, ultimately, impede the muscles' repair process and the ability to recover from strenuous exercise.

Any one of these factors can greatly increase the chances of becoming injured. Together they present a package that includes muscular discomfort, loss of performance, an increased risk of injury, and a greater likelihood of repeated injury.

How Is Flexibility Restricted?

The muscular system needs to be flexible to achieve peak performance, and stretching is the most effective way of developing and retaining flexible muscles and tendons. However, a number of other factors also contribute to a decrease in flexibility.

Flexibility, or range of movement, can be restricted by both internal and external factors. Internal factors such as bones, ligaments, muscle bulk, muscle length, tendons, and skin all restrict the amount of movement at any particular joint. As an example, the human leg cannot bend forward beyond a straight position, because of the structure of the bones and ligaments that make up the knee joint.

External factors such as age, gender, temperature, restrictive clothing, and of course any injury or disability will also have an effect on one's flexibility.

Flexibility and the Ageing Process

It is no secret that with each passing year muscles and joints seem to become stiffer and tighter. This is part of the ageing process and is caused by a combination of physical degeneration and inactivity. Although we cannot help getting older, this should not mean that we give up trying to improve our flexibility.

Age should not be a barrier to a fit and active lifestyle but certain precautions should be taken as we get older. Participants just need to work at it for longer, be a little more patient, and take a lot more care.

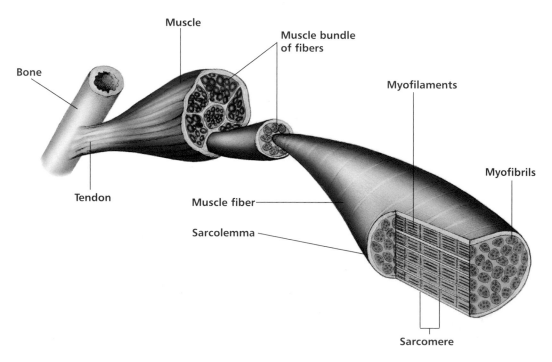

Figure 1.1: A cross-section of muscle fibers, including myofibrils, sarcomeres, and myofilaments.

Muscle Anatomy

When aiming to improve flexibility, the muscles and their fascia (sheath) should be the major focus of our flexibility training. While bones, joints, ligaments, tendons, and skin do contribute to our overall flexibility, we have very little control over these factors.

Bones and Joints

Bones and joints are structured in such a way as to allow a specific range of movement. For example, the knee joint will not allow our leg to bend any further forward past a straight leg position, no matter how hard we try.

Ligaments

Ligaments connect bone to bone and act as stabilisers for joints. Stretching the ligaments should be avoided and can result in a permanent reduction of stability at the joint, which can lead to joint weakness and injury.

Tendons

Muscles are connected to the bones by tendons, which consist of dense connective tissue. They are extremely strong yet very pliable. Tendons also play a role in joint stability and contribute less than 10% to a joint's overall flexibility; therefore tendons should not be a primary focus of stretching.

Muscles

The human body contains over 215 pairs of skeletal muscles, which make up approximately 40% of its weight. Skeletal muscles are so named because most attach to and move the skeleton, and so are responsible for movement of the body.

Skeletal muscles have an abundant supply of blood vessels and nerves, which is directly related to contraction, the primary function of skeletal muscle. Each skeletal muscle generally has one main artery to bring nutrients via the blood supply, and several veins to take away metabolic waste. The blood and nerve supply generally enters the muscle through the centre of the muscle, but occasionally toward one end, which eventually penetrates the endomysium around each muscle fiber.

The three types of skeletal muscle fiber are: red slow-twitch, intermediate fast-twitch, and white fast-twitch. The colour of each is reflected in the amount of myoglobin present, a store for oxygen. The myoglobin is able to increase the rate of oxygen diffusion, so red slow-twitch fibers are able to contract for longer periods, which is particularly useful for endurance events. The white fast-twitch fibers have a lower content of myoglobin. Because they rely on glycogen (energy) reserves, they can contract quickly, but they also fatigue quickly, so are more prevalent in sprinters, or sports where short, rapid movements are required, such as weightlifting. World-class marathon runners have been reported to possess 93–99% slow-twitch fibers in their gastrocnemius (calf) muscle, whilst world-class sprinters only possess about 25% in the same muscle (Wilmore & Costill, 1994).

Each skeletal muscle fiber is a single cylindrical muscle cell, which is surrounded by a plasma membrane called the sarcolemma. The sarcolemma features specific openings, which lead to tubes known as transverse (or T) tubules. (The sarcolemma maintains a membrane potential, which allows impulses, specifically to the sarcoplasmic reticulum (SR), to either generate or inhibit contractions.)

An individual skeletal muscle may be made up of hundreds, or even thousands, of muscle fibers bundled together and wrapped in a connective tissue sheath called the epimysium, which gives the muscle its shape, as well as providing a surface against which the surrounding muscles can move. Fascia, connective tissue outside the epimysium, surrounds and separates the muscles.

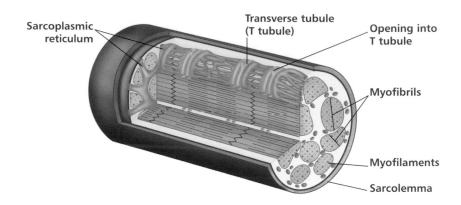

Figure 1.2: Each skeletal muscle fiber is a single cylindrical muscle cell.

Portions of the epimysium project inward to divide the muscle into compartments. Each compartment contains a bundle of muscle fibers; each of these bundles is called a fasciculus (Latin = small bundle of twigs) and is surrounded by a layer of connective tissue called the perimysium. Each fasciculus consists of a number of muscle cells, and within the fasciculus, each individual muscle cell is surrounded by the endomysium, a fine sheath of delicate connective tissue.

Skeletal muscles come in a variety of shapes, due to the arrangement of their fasciculus (English = fascicles), depending on the function of the muscle in relation to its position and action. Parallel muscles have their fasciculus running parallel to the long axis of the muscle, e.g., sartorius. Pennate muscles have short fasciculus, which are attached obliquely to the tendon, and appear feather-shaped, e.g., rectus femoris. Convergent (triangular) muscles have a broad origin with the fasciculus converging toward a single tendon, e.g., pectoralis major. Circular (sphincter) muscles have their fasciculus arranged in concentric rings around an opening, e.g., orbicularis oculi.

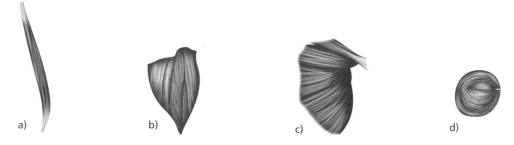

Figure 1.3: Muscle shapes: (a) parallel, (b) pennate, (c) convergent, and (d) circular.

Each muscle fiber is composed of small structures called muscle fibrils or myofibrils ("myo-" meaning "muscle" in Latin). These myofibrils lie in parallel and give the muscle cell its striated appearance, because they are composed of regularly aligned myofilaments. Myofilaments are chains of protein molecules, which under microscope appear as alternate light and dark bands. The light isotropic (I) bands are composed of the protein actin. The dark anisotropic (A) bands are composed of the protein myosin. (A third protein called titin has been identified, which accounts for about 11% of the combined muscle protein content.) When a muscle contracts, the actin filaments move between the myosin filaments, forming cross-bridges, which results in the myofibrils shortening and thickening. (See "The Physiology of Muscle Contraction.")

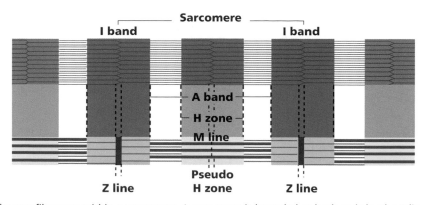

Figure 1.4: The myofilaments within a sarcomere. A sarcomere is bounded at both ends by the Z line; M line is the centre of the sarcomere; I band is composed of actin; A band is composed of myosin.

Commonly, the epimysium, perimysium, and endomysium extend beyond the fleshy part of the muscle, the belly, to form a thick ropelike tendon or broad, flat, sheet-like tendinous tissue, known as an aponeurosis. The tendon and aponeurosis form indirect attachments from muscles to the periosteum of bones or to the connective tissue of other muscles. However, more complex muscles may have multiple attachments, such as the quadriceps (four attachments). So typically a muscle spans a joint and is attached to bones by tendons at both ends. One of the bones remains relatively fixed or stable while the other end moves as a result of muscle contraction.

Each muscle fiber is innervated by a single motor nerve fiber, ending near the middle of the muscle fiber. A single motor nerve fiber and all the muscle fibers it supplies is known as a motor unit. The number of muscle fibers supplied by a single nerve fiber is dependent upon the movement required. When an exact, controlled degree of movement is required, such as in eye or finger movement, only a few muscle fibers are supplied; when a grosser movement is required, as in large muscles like gluteus maximus, several hundred fibers may be supplied.

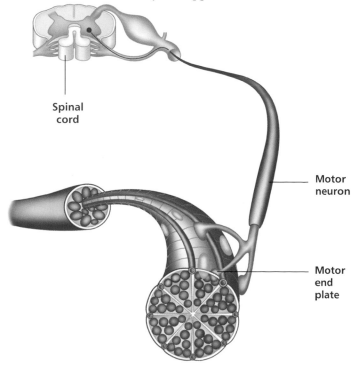

Figure 1.5: A motor unit of a skeletal muscle.

Individual skeletal muscle fibers work on an "all or nothing" principle, where stimulation of the fiber results in complete contraction of that fiber, or no contraction at all – a fiber cannot be "slightly contracted". The overall contraction of any named muscle involves the contraction of a proportion of its fibers at any one time, with others remaining relaxed.

The Physiology of Muscle Contraction

Nerve impulses cause the skeletal muscle fibers at which they terminate, to contract. The junction between a muscle fiber and the motor nerve is known as the neuromuscular junction, and this is where communication between the nerve and muscle takes place. A nerve impulse arrives at the nerve's endings, called synaptic terminals, close to the sarcolemma. These terminals contain thousands of vesicles filled with a neurotransmitter called acetylcholine (ACh). When a nerve impulse reaches the synaptic terminal, hundreds of these vesicles discharge their ACh. The ACh opens up channels, which allow sodium ions (Na+) to diffuse in. An inactive muscle fiber has a resting potential of about -95 mV. The influx of sodium ions reduces the charge, creating an end plate potential. If the end plate potential reaches the threshold voltage (approximately -50 mV), sodium ions flow in and an action potential is created within the fiber.

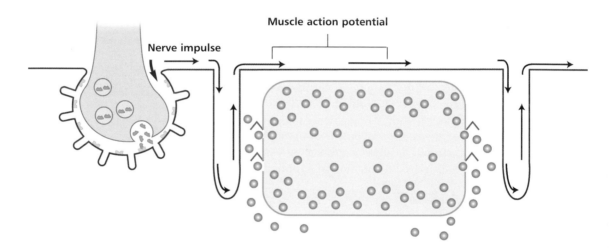

Figure 1.6: Nerve impulse triggering an action potential/muscle contraction.

No visible change occurs in the muscle fiber during (and immediately following) the action potential. This period, called the latent period, lasts from 3–10 msec. Before the latent period is over, the enzyme acetylcholinesterase breaks down the ACh in the neuromuscular junction, the sodium channels close, and the field is cleared for the arrival of another nerve impulse. The resting potential of the fiber is restored by an outflow of potassium ions. The brief period needed to restore the resting potential is called the refractory period.

So how does a muscle fiber shorten? This has been explained best by the sliding filament theory (Huxley & Hanson, 1954), which proposed that muscle fibers receive a nerve impulse (see above) that results in the release of calcium ions stored in the sarcoplasmic reticulum (SR). For muscles to work effectively, energy is required, and this is created by the breakdown of adenosine triphosphate (ATP). This energy allows the calcium ions to bind with the actin and myosin filaments to form a magnetic bond, which causes the fibers to shorten, resulting in the contraction. Muscle action continues until the calcium is depleted, at which point calcium is pumped back into the SR, where it is stored until another nerve impulse arrives.

Muscle Reflexes

Skeletal muscles contain specialized sensory units that are sensitive to muscle lengthening (stretching). These sensory units are called muscle spindles and Golgi tendon organs and they are important in detecting, responding to, and modulating changes in the length of muscle.

Muscle spindles are made up of spiral threads called intrafusal fibers, and nerve endings, both encased within a connective tissue sheath, that monitor the speed at which a muscle is lengthening. If a muscle is lengthening at speed, signals from the intrafusal fibers will fire information via the spinal cord to the nervous system so that a nerve impulse is sent back, causing the lengthening muscle to contract. The signals give continuous information to/from the muscle about position and power (proprioception).

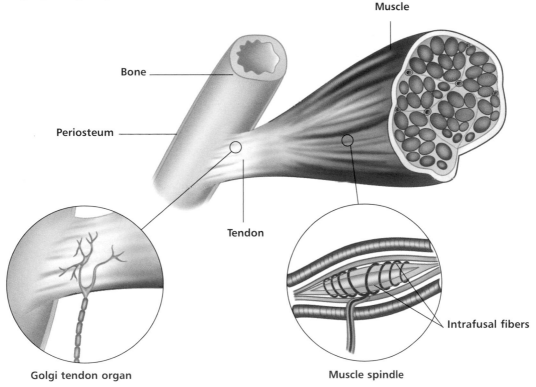

Figure 1.7: Anatomy of the muscle spindle and Golgi tendon organ.

Furthermore, when a muscle is lengthened and held, it will maintain a contractile response as long as the muscle remains stretched. This facility is known as the stretch reflex arc. Muscle spindles will remain stimulated as long as the stretch is held (see page 27).

The classic clinical example of the stretch reflex is the knee jerk test, which involves activation of the stretch receptors in the tendon, which causes reflex contraction of the muscle attached, i.e., the quadriceps.

Whereas the muscle spindles monitor the length of a muscle, the Golgi tendon organs (GTOs) in the muscle tendon are so sensitive to tension in the muscle-tendon complex, that they can respond to the contraction of a single muscle fiber. The GTOs are inhibitory in nature, performing a protective function by reducing the risk of injury. When stimulated, the GTOs inhibit the contracting (agonist) muscles and excite the antagonist muscles.

Musculo-skeletal Mechanics

Most coordinated movement involves one attachment of a skeletal muscle remaining relatively stationary, whilst the attachment at the other end moves. The proximal, more fixed attachment is known as the origin, while the attachment that lies more distally, and moves, is known as the insertion. (However, attachment is now the preferred term for origin and insertion, as it acknowledges that muscles often work so that either end can be fixed whilst the other end moves.)

Most movements require the application of muscle force, which often is accomplished by agonists (or prime movers), which are primarily responsible for movement and provide most of the force required for movement; antagonists, which have to lengthen to allow for the movement produced by the prime movers, and play a protective role; and synergists (more specifically referred to as stabilisers), which assist prime movers, and are sometimes involved in fine-tuning the direction of movement. A simple example is the flexion of the elbow, which requires shortening of the brachialis and biceps brachii (prime movers) and the relaxation of the triceps brachii (antagonist). The brachioradialis acts as the synergist by assisting the brachialis and biceps brachii.

Muscle movement can be broken down into three types of contractions: concentric, eccentric, and static (isometric). In many activities, such as running, Pilates, and yoga, all three types of contraction may occur to produce smooth, coordinated movement.

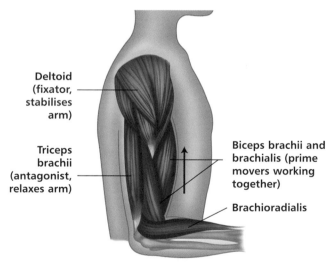

Deltoid (fixator, stabilises arm)

Triceps brachii (antagonist, relaxes arm)

Biceps brachii and brachialis (prime movers working together)

Brachioradialis

Figure 1.8: Flexion of the elbow, where brachialis and biceps brachii act as the prime movers, triceps brachii as the antagonist, and brachioradialis as the synergist.

Skeletal muscles can be broadly classified into two types:

1. Stabilisers*, which essentially stabilize a joint. They are made up of slow-twitch fibers for endurance, and assist with postural holding. They can be further subdivided into primary stabilisers, which have very deep attachments, lying close to the axis of rotation of the joint; and secondary stabilisers, which are powerful muscles, with an ability to absorb large amounts of force. Stabilisers work against gravity, and tend to become weak and long over time (Norris, 1998). Examples include multifidus, transversus abdominis (primary), and gluteus maximus and adductor magnus (secondary).

Importantly, all skeletal muscles are stabilisers and mobilisers – it depends on the movement and position of the body as to how the muscles are reacting at the time.

2. Mobilisers* are responsible for movement. They tend to be more superficial although less powerful than stabilisers, but produce a wider range of motion. They tend to cross two joints, and are made of fast-twitch fibers that produce power but lack endurance. Mobilisers assist with rapid or ballistic movement and produce high force. With time and use, they tend to tighten and shorten. Examples include the hamstrings, piriformis, and rhomboids.

A muscle's principle action, shortening, where the muscle attachments move closer together, is referred to as a concentric contraction. Because joint movement is produced, concentric contractions are also considered dynamic contractions. An example is that of holding an object, where the biceps brachii contracts concentrically, the elbow joint flexes, and the hand moves up toward the shoulder.

A movement is considered to be an eccentric contraction where the muscle may exert force while lengthening. As with concentric contraction, because joint movement is produced, this is also referred to as a dynamic contraction. The actin filaments are pulled further from the centre of the sarcomere, effectively stretching it.

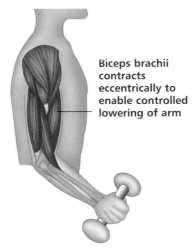

Biceps brachii contracts eccentrically to enable controlled lowering of arm

Figure 1.9: An example of eccentric contraction is the action of the biceps brachii when the elbow is extended to lower a heavy weight. Here, biceps brachii is controlling the movement by gradually lengthening in order to resist gravity.

When a muscle acts without moving, force is generated but its length remains unchanged. This is known as static (isometric) contraction.

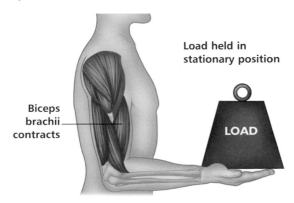

Load held in stationary position

Biceps brachii contracts

LOAD

Figure 1.10: An example of static (isometric) contraction, where a heavy weight is held, with the elbow stationary and bent at 90 degrees.

Levers

A lever is a device for transmitting (but not creating force) and consists of a rigid bar moving about a fixed point (fulcrum). More specifically, a lever consists of an effort force, resistance force, rigid bar, and a fulcrum. The bones, joints, and muscles together form a system of levers in the body, where the joints act as the fulcrum, the muscles apply the effort, and the bones carry the weight of the body part to be moved. Levers are classified according to the position of the fulcrum, resistance (load), and effort relative to each other.

In a first-class lever, the effort and resistance are located on opposite sides of the fulcrum. In a second-class lever, the effort and the resistance are located on the same side of the fulcrum, and the resistance is between the fulcrum and effort. Finally, in a third-class lever, the effort and resistance are located on the same side of the fulcrum, but the effort acts between the fulcrum and the resistance, and this is the most common type of lever in the human body.

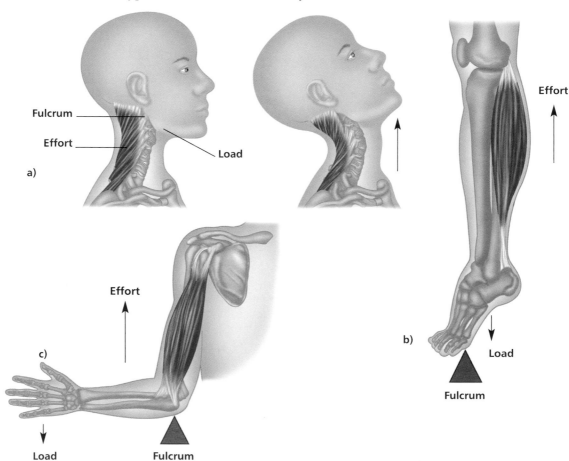

Figure 1.11: Examples of levers in the human body: (a) first-class lever, (b) second-class lever, and (c) third-class lever.

Generation of Force

The strength of skeletal muscle is reflected in its ability to generate force. If a weightlifter is able to lift 75 kg, the muscles are capable of producing enough force to lift 75 kg. Even when not trying to lift a weight, the muscles must still generate enough force to move the bones to which they are attached. A number of factors are involved in this ability to generate force, including the number and type of motor units activated, the size of the muscle, and the angle of the joint.

Reciprocal Inhibition

Most movement involves the combined effort of two or more muscles, with one muscle acting as the prime mover. Most prime movers usually have a synergistic muscle to assist them. Furthermore, most skeletal muscles have one or more antagonists that perform the opposite action. A good example might be hip abduction, in which gluteus medius acts as the prime mover, with tensor fascia latae acting synergistically and the hip adductors acting as antagonists, being reciprocally inhibited by the action of the agonists.

Reciprocal inhibition (RI) is the physiological phenomenon in which there is an automatic inhibition of a muscle when its antagonist contracts. Under special circumstances both the agonist and antagonist can contract together, known as a *co-contraction*.

Now that we have a general understanding of flexibility, muscles, and muscle mechanics, let us define stretching. Stretching, as it relates to physical health and fitness, is the process of placing particular parts of the body into a position that will lengthen the muscles and associated soft tissues.

What Happens When a Muscle Is Stretched?

Upon undertaking a regular stretching program a number of changes begin to occur within the body and specifically within the muscles themselves. Other tissues that begin to adapt to the stretching process include the ligaments, tendons, fascia, skin, and scar tissue.

As discussed earlier in this chapter, the process of lengthening the muscles and thereby increasing range of movement begins within the muscles at the sarcomeres. When a particular body part is placed into a position that lengthens the muscle, the overlap between the thick and thin myofilaments begins to decrease. Once this has been achieved and all the sarcomeres are fully stretched, the muscle fiber is at its maximum resting length. At this point further stretching will help to elongate the connective tissues and muscle fascia. Additionally, G. Goldspink (1968) and P.E. Williams & G. Goldspink (1971) concluded that *"with regular stretching over time, the number of sarcomeres is thought to increase in series, with new sarcomeres added onto the end of existing myofibrils, which in turn increases the overall muscle length and range of motion."*

Terms of Anatomical Direction

Abduction	A movement away from the midline (or to return from adduction).
Adduction	A movement toward the midline (or to return from abduction).
Anatomical position	The body is upright with the arms and hands turned forward.
Anterior	Towards the front of the body (as opposed to posterior).
Circumduction	Movement in which the distal end of a bone moves in a circle, while the proximal end remains stable.
Elevation	Movement of a part of the body upwards along the frontal plane.

Eversion	To turn the sole of the foot outward.
Extension	A movement at a joint resulting in separation of two ventral surfaces (as opposed to flexion).
Flexion	A movement at a joint resulting in approximation of two ventral surfaces (as opposed to extension).
Inferior	Below or furthest away from the head.
Inversion	To turn the sole of the foot inward.
Lateral	Located away from the midline (opposite to medial).
Medial	Situated close to or at the midline of the body or organ (opposite to lateral).
Median	Centrally located, situated in the middle of the body.
Opposition	A movement specific to the saddle joint of the thumb, that enables you to touch your thumb to the tips of the fingers of the same hand.
Palmar	Anterior surface of the hand.
Plantar	The sole of the foot.
Posterior	Relating to the back or the dorsal aspect of the body (opposite to anterior).
Pronation	To turn the palm of the hand down to face the floor, or away from the anatomical and foetal positions.
Prone	Position of the body in which the ventral surface faces down (as opposed to supine).
Rotation	Move around a fixed axis.
Superficial	On or near the surface (as opposed to deep).
Superior	Above or closest to the head.
Supination	To turn the palm of the hand up to face the ceiling, or toward the anatomical and foetal positions.

2

The Principles of Stretching

The Benefits of Stretching

Stretching is a simple and effective activity that helps to enhance athletic performance, decrease the likelihood of injury, and minimize muscle soreness. But how, specifically, is this accomplished? The benefits of stretching are:

1. Improved Range of Movement

By placing particular parts of the body in certain positions, we are able to increase the length of our muscles. As a result of this, a reduction in general muscle tension is achieved and our normal range of movement is increased.

By increasing our range of movement we are increasing the distance our limbs can move before damage occurs to the muscles and tendons. For example, the muscles and tendons in the back of our legs are put under great strain when kicking a soccer ball. Therefore, the more flexible and pliable those muscles are, the further our leg can travel forward before a strain or injury occurs to them.

The benefits of an extended range of movement include increased comfort, a greater ability to move freely, and a lessening of our susceptibility to muscle and tendon strain injuries.

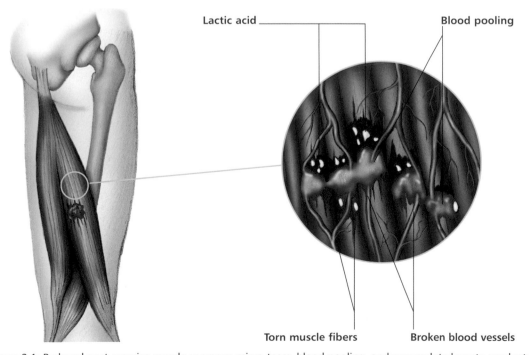

Lactic acid _____ **Blood pooling**

Torn muscle fibers **Broken blood vessels**

Figure 2.1: Reduced post-exercise muscle soreness: micro tears, blood pooling, and accumulated waste products.

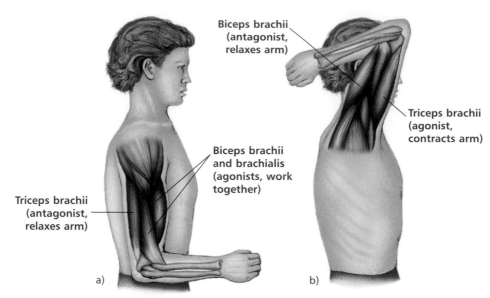

Biceps brachii
(antagonist,
relaxes arm)

Triceps brachii
(agonist,
contracts arm)

Biceps brachii
and brachialis
(agonists, work
together)

Triceps brachii
(antagonist,
relaxes arm)

a)   b)

Figure 2.2: a) a tight antagonist causing the agonist to work harder,
b) a normal interaction between agonist and antagonist.

2. Increased Power

There is a dangerous stretching myth that says, "If you stretch too much you will lose both joint stability and muscle power." This is untrue (as long as The Rules for Safe Stretching on page 25 are observed). By increasing our muscles' length we are increasing the distance over which they are able to contract. This results in a potential increase to our muscles' power and therefore increases our athletic ability, while also leading to an improvement in dynamic balance, or the ability to control our muscles.

3. Reduced Post-Exercise Muscle Soreness

We have all experienced what happens when we go for a run or to the gym for the first time in a few months. The following day our muscles are tight, sore, and stiff, and it is usually hard to even walk down a flight of stairs. This soreness that usually accompanies strenuous physical activity is often referred to as "post-exercise muscle soreness." This soreness is the result of micro tears (minute tears within the muscle fibers), blood pooling, and accumulated waste products, such as lactic acid. Stretching, as part of an effective cool-down, helps to alleviate this soreness by lengthening the individual muscle fibers, increasing blood circulation, and removing waste products.

4. Reduced Fatigue

Fatigue is a major problem for everyone, especially those who exercise: it results in a decrease in both physical and mental performance. Increased flexibility through stretching can help prevent the effects of fatigue by taking pressure off the working muscles (the agonists). For every muscle in the body there is an opposite or opposing muscle (the antagonist). If the opposing muscles are more flexible, the working muscles do not have to exert as much force against them. Therefore each movement of the working muscles actually takes less effort.

Added Benefits

Along with the benefits listed above, a regular stretching program will also help to improve posture, develop body awareness, improve coordination, promote circulation, increase energy, and improve relaxation and stress relief.

Types of Stretching

Stretching is slightly more technical than swinging a leg over a park bench. There are rules and techniques that will maximize its benefits and minimize the risk of injury. We will look at the different types of stretching, the particular benefits, and the risks and uses, as well as give a description of how each type is performed.

Just as there are many different ways to strength train, there are also many different ways to stretch. However, it is important to note that no one way in particular, or no one type of stretching, is better than another. Each type has its own advantages and disadvantages, and the key to getting the most out of stretching lies in being able to match the right type of stretching to the purpose or goal you are trying to achieve.

For example, proprioceptive neuromuscular facilitation (PNF) and passive stretching are great for creating permanent improvements in flexibility, but they are not very useful for warming up or preparing the body for activity. Dynamic stretching, on the other hand, is great for warming up, but can be dangerous if used in the initial stages of injury rehabilitation.

Although there are many different ways to stretch, they can all be grouped into one of two categories: static or dynamic.

Static Stretches

The term "static stretches" refers to stretching exercises that are performed without movement. In other words, the individual gets into the stretch position and holds the stretch for a specific amount of time. Listed below are five different types of static stretching exercises.

1. Static Stretching

Static stretching is performed by placing the body into a position whereby the muscle (or group of muscles) to be stretched is under tension. To begin, both the antagonist, or opposing muscle, and the agonist, or muscle to be stretched, are relaxed. Then slowly and cautiously the body is moved to increase the tension of the muscle being stretched. At this point the position is held or maintained to allow the muscle to lengthen.

A minimum hold time of about 20 seconds is required for the muscle to relax and start to lengthen, while diminishing returns are experienced after 45–60 seconds.

Static stretching is a very safe and effective form of stretching, with a limited threat of injury. It is a good choice for beginners and sedentary individuals.

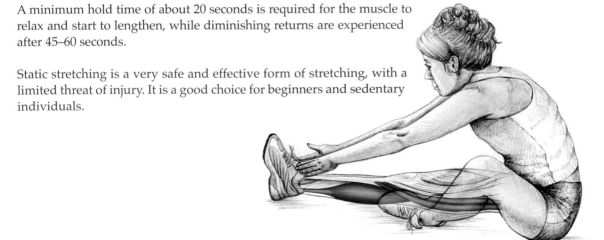

Figure 2.3: An example of static stretching.

2. Passive (or Assisted) Stretching

This form of stretching is very similar to static stretching; however, another person or apparatus is used to help further stretch the muscle. Due to the greater force applied to the muscle, this form of stretching is slightly more hazardous. Therefore, it is very important that any apparatus used is both solid and stable. When using a partner it is imperative that no jerky or bouncing force is applied to the stretched muscle. So, choose a partner carefully – the partner is responsible for the safety of the muscles and joints while performing the stretching exercises.

Passive stretching is useful in helping to attain a greater range of movement, but carries with it a slightly higher risk of injury. It can also be used effectively as part of a rehabilitation program or as part of a cool-down.

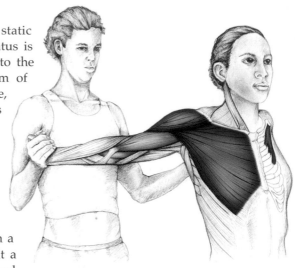

Figure 2.4: An example of passive stretching.

3. Active Stretching

Active stretching is performed without any aid or assistance from an external force. This form of stretching involves using only the strength of the opposing muscles (antagonists) to generate a stretch within the targeted muscle group (agonists). The contraction of the opposing muscles helps to relax the stretched muscles. A classic example of an active stretch is one where an individual raises one leg straight out in front as high as possible and then maintains that position without any assistance from a partner or object.

Active stretching is useful as a rehabilitation tool and a very effective form of conditioning before moving on to dynamic stretching exercises. This type of stretching exercise is usually quite difficult to hold and maintain for long periods of time and the stretch position is therefore usually only held for 10–15 seconds.

4. PNF Stretching

PNF stretching is a more advanced form of flexibility training, which involves both the stretching and contracting of the muscle group being targeted. PNF stretching was originally developed as a form of rehabilitation and for that function it is very effective. It is also excellent for targeting specific muscle groups and, as well as increasing flexibility (and range of movement), it also improves muscular strength.

There are many different variations of the PNF stretching principle and sometimes it is referred to as "contract-relax stretching" or "hold-relax stretching." Another variation of the PNF technique is "post isometric relaxation (PIR)."

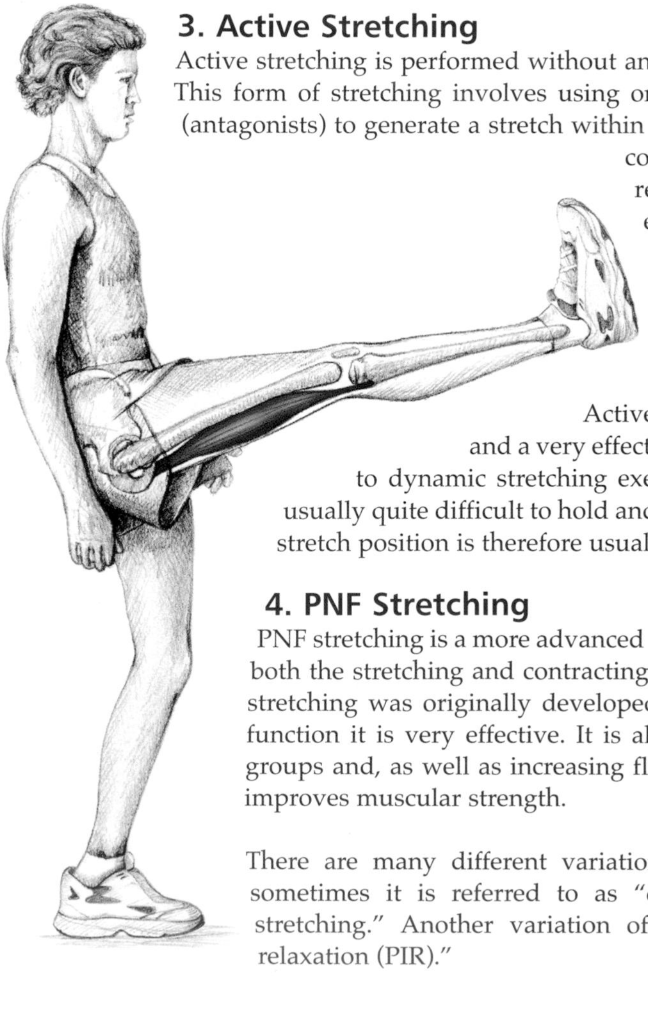

Figure 2.5: An example of active stretching.

The area to be stretched is positioned so that the muscle (or muscle group) is under tension. The individual then contracts the stretched muscle for 5–6 seconds while a partner (or immoveable object) applies sufficient resistance to inhibit movement. The effort of contraction should be relevant to the level of conditioning. The contracted muscle is then relaxed and a controlled stretch is applied for about 30 seconds. The athlete is then allowed 15 to 30 seconds to recover and the process is repeated 2–4 times.

Information differs slightly about timing recommendations for PNF stretching. Although there are conflicting responses to the questions "For how long should I contract the muscle group?" and "For how long should I rest between each stretch?", it is my professional opinion that, through a study of research literature and personal experience, the above timing recommendations provide the maximum benefits from PNF stretching.

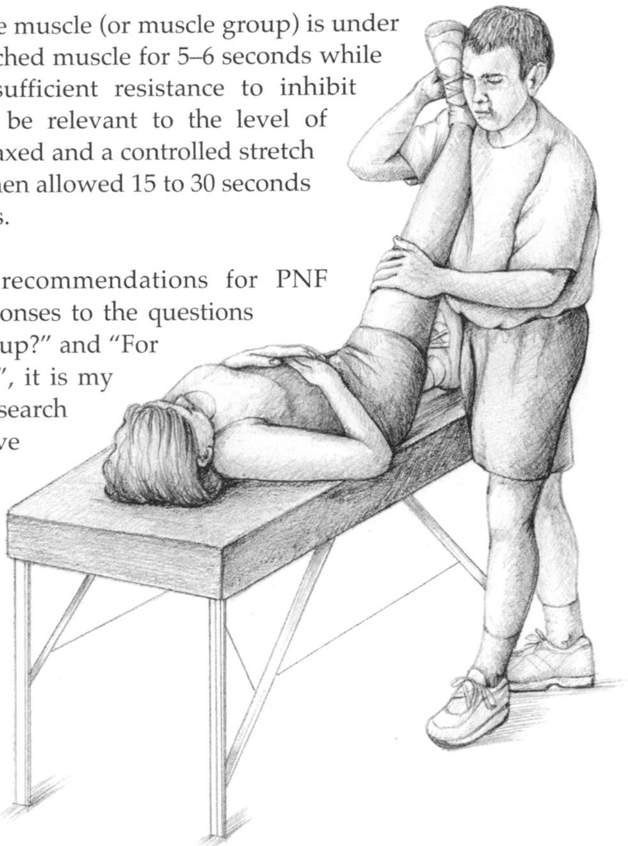

5. Isometric Stretching

Isometric stretching is a form of passive stretching similar to PNF, but the contractions are held for a longer period of time. Isometric stretching places high demands on the stretched muscles and is not recommended for children or adolescents who are still growing. Other recommendations include allowing at least 48 hours' rest between isometric stretching sessions and performing only one isometric stretching exercise per muscle group in a session.

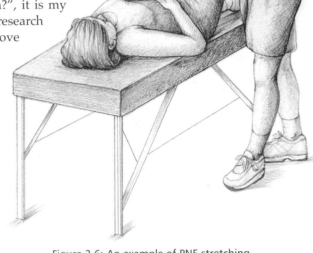

Figure 2.6: An example of PNF stretching.

A classic example of how isometric stretching is used is the standing "push-the-wall" calf stretch (see Chapter 12, Stretch J06), where the participant stands upright, leans forward against a wall, and then places one foot as far from the wall as is comfortable while making sure that the heel remains on the ground. In this position, the participant then contracts the calf muscles as if trying to push the wall down.

To perform an isometric stretch, assume the position of the passive stretch and then contract the stretched muscle for 10–15 seconds. Be sure that all movement of the limb is restricted. Then relax the muscle for at least 20 seconds. This procedure should be repeated 2–5 times.

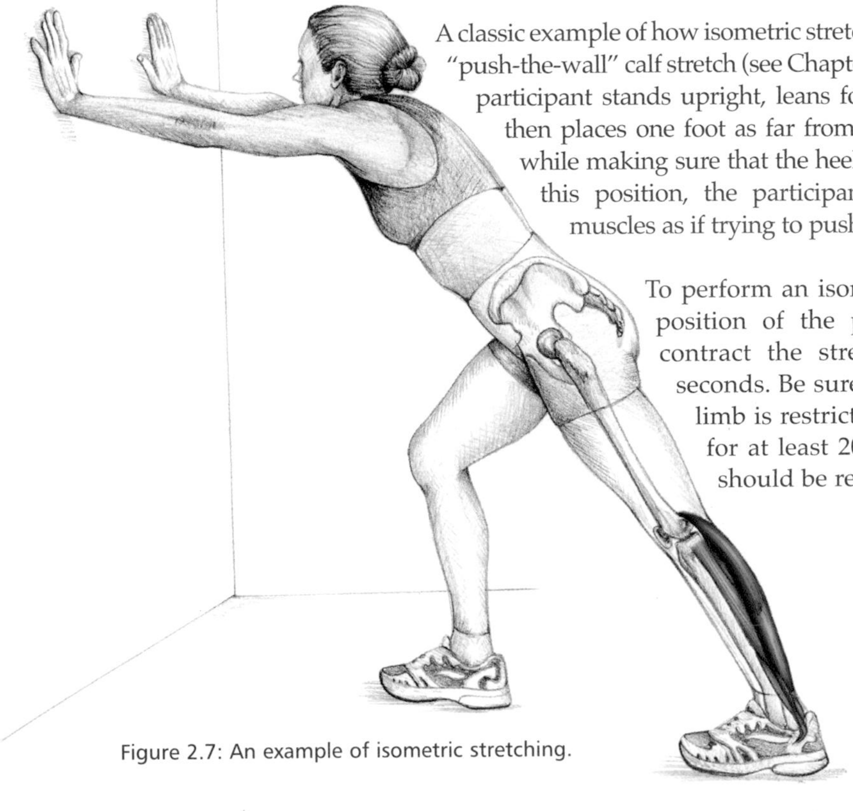

Figure 2.7: An example of isometric stretching.

Dynamic Stretches

The term "dynamic stretches" refers to stretching exercises that are performed with movement. In other words, the individual uses a swinging or bouncing motion to extend their range of movement and flexibility. Listed below are four different types of dynamic stretching exercises.

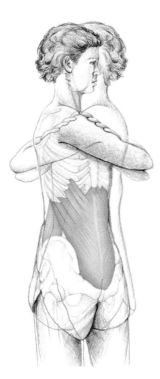

1. Ballistic Stretching

Ballistic stretching is an outdated form of stretching that uses momentum generated by rapid swinging, bouncing, and rebounding movements to force a body part past its normal range of movement.

The risks associated with ballistic stretching far outweigh the gains, especially when better gains can be achieved by using other forms like dynamic and PNF stretching. Other than potential injury, the main disadvantage of ballistic stretching is that it fails to allow the stretched muscles time to adapt to the stretched position and, instead, may cause the muscles to tighten up by repeatedly triggering the stretch (or myotatic) reflex (see page 27).

2. Dynamic Stretching

Unlike ballistic stretching, dynamic stretching uses a controlled, soft bounce or swinging motion to move a particular body part to the limit of its range of movement. The force of the bounce or swing is gradually increased but should never become radical or uncontrolled.

Do not confuse dynamic stretching with ballistic stretching. Dynamic stretching is slow, gentle, and very purposeful. At no time during dynamic stretching should a body part be forced past the joint's normal range of movement. Ballistic stretching, on the other hand, is much more aggressive and its very purpose is to force the body part beyond the limit of its normal range of movement.

Figure 2.8: An example of ballistic stretching.

3. Active Isolated Stretching

Active isolated (AI) stretching is a new form of stretching developed by Aaron L. Mattes and is sometimes referred to as the "Mattes Method." It works by contracting the antagonists, or opposing muscle group, which forces the stretched muscle group to relax. The procedure for performing AI stretching is as follows.

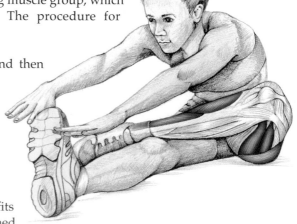

1. Choose the muscle group to be stretched and then assume the appropriate starting position.
2. Actively contract the antagonists, or opposing muscle group.
3. Move into the stretch quickly and smoothly.
4. Hold for 1–2 seconds and then release the stretch.
5. Repeat 5–10 times.

While AI stretching certainly has some benefits (mainly for the professional or well-conditioned athlete), it also has a lot of unsubstantiated claims. One such claim is that AI stretching does not engage the stretch reflex, because the stretch is only held for

Figure 2.9: An example of active isolated stretching.

2 seconds or less (Mattes 2000; Wharton 1996). This, however, defies basic muscle physiology. The stretch reflex in the calf muscle, for example, is triggered within three-hundredths of a second, so any claim that AI stretching can somehow bypass or outsmart the stretch reflex is nothing more than wishful thinking.

4. Resistance Stretching and Loaded Stretching

Resistance stretching and loaded stretching are forms of dynamic stretching that both contract and lengthen a muscle at the same time. They work by stretching a muscle group through its entire range of motion while under contraction. For this reason, both resistance stretching and loaded stretching are as much about strengthening a muscle group as they are about stretching it.

Like AI stretching above, resistance stretching and loaded stretching do have their benefits. The five-time Olympic swimmer Dara Torres credits a portion of her swimming success to the use of resistance stretching. However, these forms of stretching place high demands on the musculoskeletal system and therefore are recommended only for professional or well-conditioned athletes.

The Rules for Safe Stretching

As with most activities there are rules and guidelines to ensure that they are safe. Stretching is no exception – it can be extremely dangerous and harmful if done incorrectly. It is vitally important that the following rules be adhered to, both for safety and for maximizing the potential benefits of stretching.

There is often confusion and concern about which stretches are good and which stretches are bad. In most cases someone has told the inquirer that they should not do this stretch or that stretch, or that this is a good stretch and that is a bad stretch.

Are there only good stretches and bad stretches? Is there no middle ground? And if there are only good and bad stretches, how do we decide which ones are good and which ones are bad?

There is no such thing as a good or bad stretch!

Just as there are no good or bad exercises, there are no good or bad stretches: only what is appropriate for the specific requirements of the individual. So a stretch that is perfectly okay for one person may not be okay for someone else.

Let me use an example. A person with a shoulder injury would not be expected to do push-ups or freestyle swimming, but that does not mean that these are bad exercises. Now, consider the same scenario from a stretching point of view. That same person should avoid shoulder stretches, but that does not mean that all shoulder stretches are bad.

The stretch itself is neither good nor bad. It is the way the stretch is performed and by whom it is being performed that makes stretching either effective and safe, or ineffective and harmful. To place a particular stretch into a category of "good" or "bad" is foolish and dangerous. To label a stretch as "good" gives people the impression that they can do that stretch whenever and however they want and it will not cause them any problems.

The specific requirements of the individual are what is important!

Remember, stretches are neither good nor bad. However, when choosing a stretch there are a number of precautions and "checks" we need to perform before giving that stretch the okay.

1. Firstly, make a general review of the individual. Are they healthy and physically active, or have they been leading a sedentary lifestyle for the past 5 years? Are they a professional athlete? Are they recovering from a serious injury? Do they have aches, pains, or muscle and joint stiffness in any area of their body?

2. Secondly, make a specific review of the area, or muscle group, to be stretched. Are the muscles healthy? Is there any damage to the joints, ligaments, tendons, etc.? Has the area been injured recently, or is it still recovering from an injury?

If the muscle group being stretched is not 100% healthy, avoid stretching this area altogether. Work on recovery and rehabilitation before moving on to specific stretching exercises. If, however, the individual is healthy and the area to be stretched is free from injury, then apply the following to all stretches.

1. Warm Up Prior to Stretching

This first rule is often overlooked and can lead to serious injury if not performed effectively. Trying to stretch muscles that have not been warmed is like trying to stretch old, dry rubber bands: they may snap.

Warming up prior to stretching does a number of beneficial things, but primarily its purpose is to prepare the body and mind for more strenuous activity. One of the ways it achieves this is by helping to increase the body's core temperature while also increasing the body's muscle temperature. By increasing muscle temperature we are helping to make the muscles loose, supple, and pliable. This is essential to ensure the maximum benefit is gained from our stretching.

The correct warm-up also has the effect of increasing both our heart rate and our respiratory rate. This increases blood flow, which in turn increases the delivery of oxygen and nutrients to the working muscles. All this helps to prepare the muscles for stretching.

A correct warm-up should consist of light physical activity. Both the intensity and duration of the warm-up (or how hard and how long) should be governed by the fitness level of the participating athlete, although a correct warm-up for most people should take about 10 minutes and result in a light sweat.

2. Stretch Before and After Exercise

The question often arises: "Should I stretch before or after exercise?" This is not an either/or situation: both are essential. It is no good stretching after exercise and counting that as our pre-exercise stretch for next time. Stretching after exercise has a totally different purpose to stretching before exercise. The two are not the same.

The purpose of stretching before exercise is to help prevent injury. Stretching does this by lengthening the muscles and tendons, which in turn increases our range of movement. This ensures that we are able to move freely without restriction or injury occurring.

However, stretching after exercise has a very different role. Its purpose is primarily to aid in the repair and recovery of the muscles and tendons. By lengthening the muscles and tendons, stretching helps to prevent tight muscles and delayed muscle soreness that usually accompanies strenuous exercise.

After exercise, our stretching should be done as part of a cool-down. The cool-down will vary depending on the duration and intensity of exercise undertaken, but will usually consist of 5–10 minutes of very light physical activity and be followed by 5–10 minutes of static stretching exercises.

An effective cool-down involving light physical activity and stretching will help to rid waste products from the muscles, prevent blood pooling, and promote the delivery of oxygen and nutrients to the muscles. All this assists in returning the body to a pre-exercise level, thus aiding the recovery process.

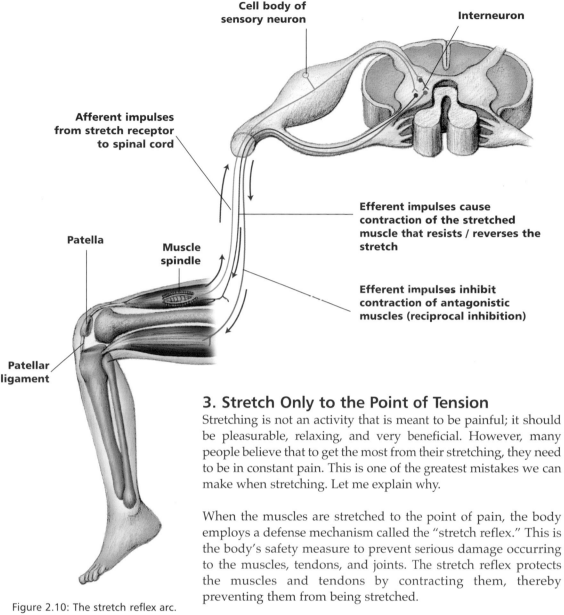

Cell body of sensory neuron

Interneuron

Afferent impulses from stretch receptor to spinal cord

Efferent impulses cause contraction of the stretched muscle that resists / reverses the stretch

Patella

Muscle spindle

Efferent impulses inhibit contraction of antagonistic muscles (reciprocal inhibition)

Patellar ligament

Figure 2.10: The stretch reflex arc.

3. Stretch Only to the Point of Tension

Stretching is not an activity that is meant to be painful; it should be pleasurable, relaxing, and very beneficial. However, many people believe that to get the most from their stretching, they need to be in constant pain. This is one of the greatest mistakes we can make when stretching. Let me explain why.

When the muscles are stretched to the point of pain, the body employs a defense mechanism called the "stretch reflex." This is the body's safety measure to prevent serious damage occurring to the muscles, tendons, and joints. The stretch reflex protects the muscles and tendons by contracting them, thereby preventing them from being stretched.

So to avoid the stretch reflex, avoid pain. Never push the stretch beyond what is comfortable. Only stretch to the point where tension can be felt in the muscles. This way, injury will be avoided and the maximum benefits from stretching will be achieved.

4. Stretch All Major Muscles and Their Opposing Muscle Groups

When stretching, it is vitally important that we pay attention to all the major muscle groups in the body. Just because a particular sport may place a lot of emphasis on the legs, for example, that does not mean that one can neglect the muscles of the upper body in a stretching routine.

All the muscles play an important part in any physical activity, not just a select few. Muscles in the upper body, for example, are extremely important in any running sport. They play a vital role in the stability and balance of the body during the running motion. Therefore it is important to keep them both flexible and supple.

Every muscle in the body has an opposing muscle that acts against it. For example, the muscles in the front of the leg (the quadriceps) are opposed by the muscles in the back of the leg (the hamstrings). These two groups of muscles provide a resistance to each other to balance the body. If one of these groups of muscles becomes stronger or more flexible than the other group, it is likely to lead to imbalances that can result in injury or postural problems. For example, hamstring tears are a common injury in most running sports. They are often caused by strong quadriceps and weak, inflexible hamstrings. This imbalance puts a great deal of pressure on the hamstrings and can result in a muscle tear or strain.

5. Stretch Gently and Slowly

Stretching gently and slowly helps to relax our muscles, which in turn makes stretching more pleasurable and beneficial. This will also help to avoid muscle tears and strains that can be caused by rapid, jerky movements.

6. Breathe Slowly and Easily While Stretching

Many people unconsciously hold their breath while stretching. This causes tension in our muscles, which in turn makes it very difficult to stretch. To avoid this, remember to breathe slowly and deeply during all stretching exercises. This helps to relax our muscles, promote blood flow, and increase the delivery of oxygen and nutrients to our muscles.

An Example

By taking a look at one of the most controversial stretches ever performed, we can see how the above rules are applied. The stretch pictured below causes many a person to go into complete meltdown. It has a reputation as a dangerous, bad stretch and should be avoided at all costs.

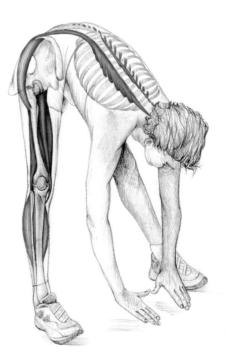

So why is it that at every Olympic Games, Commonwealth Games, and World Championships, sprinters can be seen doing this stretch before their events? Let us apply the above checks to find out.

Firstly, consider the person performing the stretch. Are they healthy, fit, and physically active? If not, this is not a stretch they should be doing. Are they elderly, overweight, or unfit? Are they young and still growing? Do they lead a sedentary lifestyle? If so, they should avoid this stretch! This first consideration alone would prohibit 50% of the population from doing this stretch.

Secondly, review the area to be stretched. This stretch obviously puts a large strain on the muscles of the hamstrings and lower back. So if our hamstrings or lower back are not

Figure 2.11: Controversial stretch?

100% healthy, we are not to perform this stretch. This second consideration would probably rule out another 25%, which means this stretch is only suitable for about 25% of the population – or, the well-trained, physically fit, injury-free athlete.

Then apply the six precautions above and the well-trained, physically fit, injury-free athlete can perform this stretch safely and effectively.

Remember, the stretch itself is neither good nor bad. It is the way the stretch is performed and by whom it is being performed that makes stretching either effective and safe, or ineffective and harmful.

How to Stretch Properly

1. When to Stretch

Stretching needs to be as important as the rest of our training. If we are involved in any competitive type of sport or exercise then it is crucial that we make time for specific stretching workouts. Set time aside to work on particular areas that are tight or stiff. The more involved and committed we are to our exercise and fitness, the more time and effort we will need to commit to stretching.

As discussed earlier it is important to stretch both before and after exercise. But when else should we stretch and what type of stretching is best for a particular purpose?

Choosing the right type of stretching for the right purpose will make a big difference to the effectiveness of our flexibility program. Here are some suggestions for when to use the different types of stretches.

For warming up, dynamic stretching is the most effective, while for cooling-down, static, passive, or PNF stretching is best. For improving range of movement, try PNF and active isolated stretching; for rehabilitation, a combination of PNF, isometric, and active stretching will give the best results.

So when else should we stretch? Stretch periodically throughout the entire day. It is a great way to keep loose and to help ease the stress of everyday life. One of the most productive ways to utilize our time is to stretch while we are watching television. Start with 5 minutes of marching or jogging on the spot then take a seat on the floor in front of the television and start stretching.

Competition is a time when great demands are placed on the body; it is therefore vitally important that we are in peak physical condition. Our flexibility should be at its best just before competition. Too many injuries are caused by the sudden exertion that is needed for any sort of competitive sport. Get strict on stretching before competition.

2. Hold, Count, Repeat

For how long should I hold each stretch? How often should I stretch? For how long should I stretch?

These are the most commonly asked questions when discussing the topic of stretching. Although there are conflicting responses to these questions, it is my professional opinion that, through a study of research literature and personal experience, what follows is currently the most correct and beneficial information.

"For how long should I hold each stretch?" This question causes the most conflict. Some text will tell us that as little as 10 seconds is enough. This is a bare minimum: 10 seconds is only just enough time for the muscles to relax and start to lengthen. For any real benefit to our flexibility we should hold each stretch for at least 20–30 seconds.

The time we commit to our stretching will be relative to our level of involvement in our particular sport. So, for people looking to increase their general level of health and fitness, a minimum of about 20 seconds will be enough. However, if we are involved in high-level competitive sport we need to hold each stretch for at least 30 seconds and start to extend that to 60 seconds and beyond.

"How often should I stretch?" This same principle of adjusting our level of commitment to our level of involvement in our sport applies to the number of times we should stretch each muscle group. For example, the beginner should stretch each muscle group 2–3 times. However, if we are involved at a more advanced level in our sport we should stretch each muscle group 3–5 times.

"For how long should I stretch?" Again, the same principle applies. For the beginner, about 5–10 minutes is enough, and for the professional athlete, anything up to two hours. If we feel that we are somewhere between the beginner and the professional, we should adjust the time we spend stretching accordingly.

Please do not be impatient with stretching. Nobody can get fit in a couple of weeks, so do not expect miracles from a stretching routine. Looking long term, some muscle groups may need a minimum of three months of intense stretching to see any real improvement. So stick with it – it is well worth the effort.

3. Sequence

When starting a stretching program it is a good idea to start with a general range of stretches for the entire body, instead of just a select few. The idea of this is to reduce overall muscle tension and to increase the mobility of our joints and limbs.

The next step should be to increase overall flexibility by starting to extend the muscles and tendons beyond their normal range of movement. Following this, we work on specific areas that are tight or important for our particular sport. Remember, all this takes time. This sequence of stretches may take up to three months for us to see real improvement, especially if we have no background in agility-based activities or are heavily muscled.

No data exists on what order we should do our stretches in. However, it is recommended that we start with sitting stretches, because there is less chance of injury while sitting, before moving on to standing stretches. To make it easier we may want to start with the ankles and move up to the neck, or vice-versa. It really does not matter as long as we cover all the major muscle groups and their opposing muscles.

Once we have advanced beyond improving our overall flexibility and are working on improving the range of movement of specific muscles, or muscle groups, it is important to isolate those muscles during our stretching routines. To do this, concentrate on only one muscle group at a time. For example, instead of trying to stretch the hamstrings of both legs at the same time, concentrate on the hamstrings of only one leg at a time. Stretching this way will help to reduce the resistance from other supporting muscle groups.

4. Posture

Posture, or alignment, while stretching is one of the most neglected aspects of flexibility training. It is important to be aware of how crucial it can be to the overall benefits of our stretching. Bad posture and incorrect technique can cause imbalances in the muscles that can lead to injury, while proper posture will ensure that the targeted muscle group receives the best possible stretch.

In many instances a major muscle group can be made up of a number of different muscles. If our posture is sloppy or incorrect, certain stretching exercises may put more emphasis on one particular muscle in that muscle group, thus causing an imbalance that could lead to injury.

For example, when stretching the hamstrings it is imperative that we keep both feet pointing straight up. If our feet fall to one side, this will put undue stress on one particular part of the hamstrings, which could result in a muscle imbalance.

How to Use Stretching as Part of the Warm-up

Lately, I have been receiving a lot of questions regarding the latest studies and research findings on stretching, and the most popular question that is asked concerns the role that stretching plays as part of the warm-up procedure.

Currently, there seems to be a lot of confusion about how and when stretching should be used as part of the warm-up, and some people are under the impression that stretching should be avoided altogether.

This is a very important issue and needs to be clarified. The following information is provided to dispel some common myths and misconceptions about stretching and its role as part of the warm-up procedure.

What has science got to say?

Most of the studies I have reviewed attempt to determine the effects of stretching on injury prevention. This is a mistake in itself and shows a lack of understanding as to how stretching is used as part of an injury prevention program and the warm-up.

Stretching and its effect on physical performance and injury prevention is something that just cannot be measured scientifically. Certainly you can measure the effect of stretching on flexibility with simple tests like the Sit and Reach test, but then to determine how that affects athletic performance or injury susceptibility is very difficult, if not near impossible.

One of the more recent studies on stretching supports this view by stating that: Due to the paucity, heterogeneity, and poor quality of the available studies no definitive conclusions can be drawn as to the value of stretching for reducing the risk of exercise-related injury. (Weldon 2003)

To put the above quote in layman's terms, there have not been enough studies done and the ones that have been are not specific or consistent enough.

The greatest misconception

Confusion about what stretching accomplishes as part of the warm-up procedure is causing many to abandon stretching altogether. The key to understanding the role stretching plays can be found in the previous sentence – but you have to read it carefully.

Stretching . . . as part of the warm-up!

Here is the key: stretching is a critical part of the warm-up, but it is not the warm-up.

Do not make the mistake of thinking that doing a few stretches constitutes a warm-up. An effective warm-up has a number of very important key elements that work together to minimize the likelihood of sports injury and prepare the individual for physical activity.

Identifying the components of an effective and safe warm-up, and executing them in the correct order, is critical. Remember, stretching is only one part of an effective warm-up, and its place in the warm-up procedure is specific and dependent on the other components.

The four key elements that should be included to ensure an effective and complete warm-up procedure are:

1. **The general warm-up:** This phase consists of 5 to 15 minutes of light physical activity. The aim here is to elevate the heart rate and respiratory rate, increase blood flow, and increase muscle temperature.

2. **Static stretching:** Next, 5 to 10 minutes of gentle static stretching should be incorporated into the general warm-up to gradually lengthen all the muscles of the major muscle groups and associated soft tissues of the body.

3. **The sports-specific warm-up:** During this phase, 10 to 15 minutes of sport-specific drills and exercises should be used to prepare the athlete for the specific demands of their chosen sport.

4. **Dynamic stretching:** This component involves a controlled, soft bounce or swinging motion to move a particular body part to the limit of its range of movement. The force of the bounce or swing is gradually increased but should never become extreme or uncontrolled.

All four parts of the warm-up are equally important and any one part should not be neglected or thought of as not necessary. The four elements work together to bring the body and mind to a physical peak, ensuring that the athlete is prepared for the activity to come.

Please note the following three points:

1. Dynamic stretching carries with it an increased risk of injury if used incorrectly.

2. The time recommendations given in the above warm-up procedure relate specifically to the requirements of a serious athlete. Adjust the times accordingly if your athletic participation is not at a professional level.

3. Recent studies have shown that static stretching may have an adverse effect on muscle contraction speed and therefore impair performance of athletes involved in sports requiring high levels of power and speed. It is for this reason that static stretching is conducted early in the warm-up and is always followed by sports-specific drills and dynamic stretching.

What conclusions can we make?

Stretching is beneficial when used correctly. Remember, stretching is just one very important component that assists in reducing the risk of injury and improving athletic performance. The best results are achieved when stretching is used in combination with other injury reduction techniques and conditioning exercises.

3

Neck and Shoulders

The neck and shoulders are comprised of a multitude of muscles that control the head and upper arm. The muscles around the neck and shoulders, along with the structure of the joints, allow for a large range of movement, including: flexion; extension; hyperextension; lateral flexion; adduction; abduction; and rotation. The lateral vertebral muscles of the neck comprise the **scalenes** group, which run from the transverse processes of the cervical vertebrae downward to the ribs, plus **sternocleidomastoideus**, a long strap muscle with two heads. The **platysma** is the muscle that may be seen to stand out, for example, in a runner finishing a hard race.

Deltoideus is composed of three parts; anterior, middle, and posterior. Only the middle part is multipennate, probably because its mechanical disadvantage of abduction of the shoulder joint requires extra strength. It acts as a shock absorber, protecting the shoulder from impact. **Trapezius** is a major mover of the shoulder; the left and right trapezius viewed as a whole create a trapezium in shape, thus giving this muscle its name. **Levator scapulae** is deep to sternocleidomastoideus and trapezius, and is named after its action of elevating the scapula. The **serratus anterior** forms the medial wall of the axilla, the region between the upper thoracic wall and the upper limb, along with the upper five ribs. It is a large muscle composed of a series of finger-like slips.

The rotator cuff is a collection of muscles that comprises of **supraspinatus**, **infraspinatus**, **teres minor**, and **subscapularis**; they act to hold the "ball" of the shoulder balanced in the right position in the "socket" of the scapula during movements of the shoulder, thus helping to prevent dislocation of the joint. The subscapularis constitutes the greater part of the posterior wall of the axilla, along with **teres major**, and the tendon of latissimus dorsi, which passes around it.

Erector spinae, also called sacrospinalis, comprises three sets of muscles organised in parallel columns. From lateral to medial, they are: iliocostalis, longissimus, and spinalis. Longissimus is the intermediate part of the erector spinae. It may be subdivided into thoracis, cervicis, and capitis portions. The spinalis is the most medial part of the erector spinae. It may also be subdivided into thoracis, cervicis, and capitis portions. The **transversospinalis** muscles are a composite of three small muscle groups situated deep to erector spinae. However, unlike erector spinae, each group lies successively deeper from the surface rather than side-by-side. The muscle groups are, from more superficial to deep: semispinalis, multifidus, and rotatores. Their fibers generally extend upward and medially from transverse processes to higher spinous processes. Multifidus and rotatores are discussed in Chapter 6.

Sports that benefit from these neck and shoulder stretches include: archery; batting sports like cricket, baseball, and softball; boxing; contact sports like soccer, American football (gridiron), and rugby; golf; racquet sports like tennis, badminton, and squash; swimming; throwing sports like cricket, baseball, and field events; wrestling.

A01: LATERAL NECK STRETCH

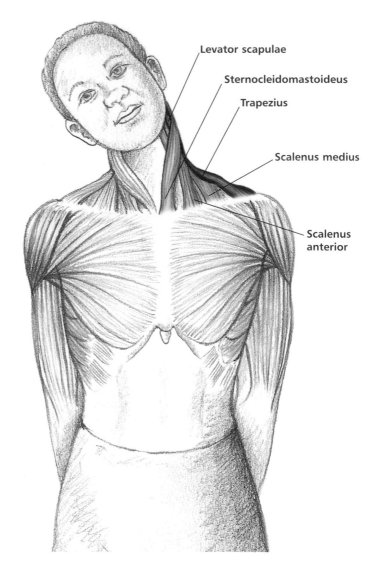

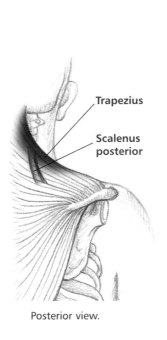

Trapezius

Scalenus posterior

Posterior view.

Levator scapulae

Sternocleidomastoideus

Trapezius

Scalenus medius

Scalenus anterior

Technique
Look forward while keeping your head up. Slowly move your ear towards your shoulder while keeping your hands behind your back.

Muscles being stretched
Primary muscles: Levator scapulae. Trapezius. Secondary muscles: Sternocleidomastoideus. Scalenus anterior, medius and posterior.

Sports that benefit from this stretch
Boxing. American football (gridiron). Rugby. Swimming. Wrestling.

Sports injury where stretch may be useful
Neck muscle strain. Whiplash (neck sprain). Cervical nerve stretch syndrome. Wryneck (acute torticollis).

Additional information for performing this stretch correctly
Keep your shoulders down and your hands behind your back. Do not lift your shoulders up when you tilt your head to the side.

Complementary stretch
A02.

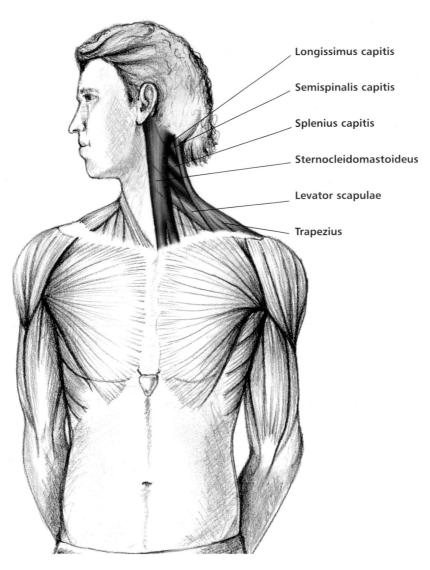

- Longissimus capitis
- Semispinalis capitis
- Splenius capitis
- Sternocleidomastoideus
- Levator scapulae
- Trapezius

Technique
Stand upright while keeping your shoulders still and your head up. Slowly rotate your chin towards your shoulder.

Muscles being stretched
Primary muscles: Sternocleidomastoideus. Splenius capitis. Semispinalis capitis. Longissimus capitis.
Secondary muscles: Levator scapulae. Trapezius.

Sports that benefit from this stretch
Archery. Boxing. American football (gridiron). Rugby. Swimming. Wrestling.

Sports injury where stretch may be useful
Neck muscle strain. Whiplash (neck sprain). Cervical nerve stretch syndrome. Wryneck (acute torticollis).

Additional information for performing this stretch correctly
Keep your head up. Do not let your chin fall towards your shoulders.

Complementary stretch
A06.

A03: FORWARD FLEXION NECK STRETCH

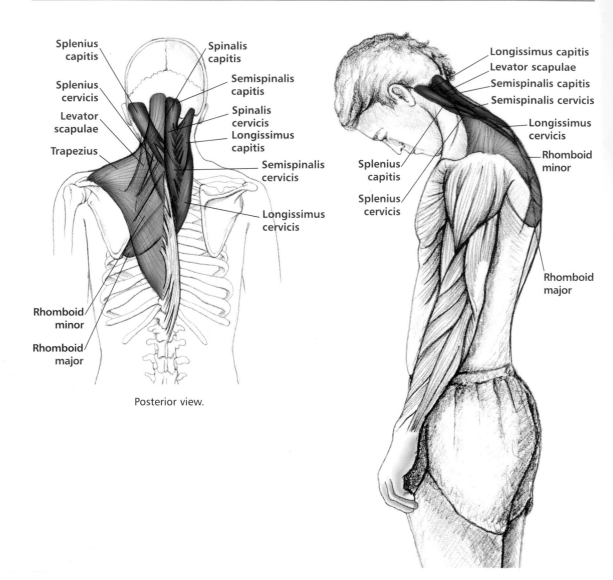

Posterior view.

Technique
Stand upright and let your chin fall forward towards your chest. Relax your shoulders and keep your hands by your side.

Muscles being stretched
Primary muscles: Semispinalis capitis and cervicis. Spinalis capitis and cervicis. Longissimus capitis and cervicis. Splenius capitis and cervicis.
Secondary muscles: Levator scapulae. Trapezius. Rhomboids.

Sports that benefit from this stretch
Boxing. American football (gridiron). Rugby. Cycling. Swimming. Wrestling.

Sports injury where stretch may be useful
Neck muscle strain. Whiplash (neck sprain). Cervical nerve stretch syndrome. Wryneck (acute torticollis).

Common problems and more information for performing this stretch correctly
Some people are more flexible in the upper back and neck than others. Do not overstretch by forcing your head down: instead, relax and let the weight of your head do the stretching for you.

Complementary stretch
A07.

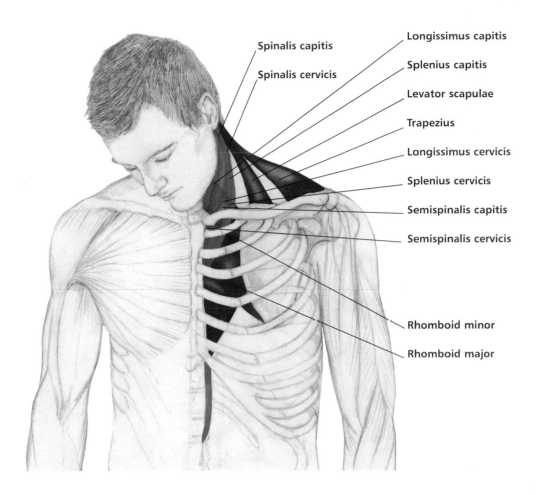

Spinalis capitis

Spinalis cervicis

Longissimus capitis

Splenius capitis

Levator scapulae

Trapezius

Longissimus cervicis

Splenius cervicis

Semispinalis capitis

Semispinalis cervicis

Rhomboid minor

Rhomboid major

Technique
Stand upright and let your chin fall forward towards your chest. Then gently lean your head to one side. Relax your shoulders and keep your hands by your side.

Muscles being stretched
Primary muscles: Levator scapulae. Trapezius. Rhomboids.
Secondary muscles: Semispinalis capitis and cervicis. Spinalis capitis and cervicis. Longissimus capitis and cervicis. Splenius capitis and cervicis.

Sports that benefit from this stretch
Archery. Boxing. Soccer. American football (gridiron). Rugby. Cycling. Golf. Swimming. Wrestling.

Sports injury where stretch may be useful
Neck muscle strain. Whiplash (neck sprain). Cervical nerve stretch syndrome. Wryneck (acute torticollis).

Common problems and more information for performing this stretch correctly
Some people are more flexible in the upper back and neck than others. Do not overstretch by forcing your head down; instead, relax and let the weight of your head do the stretching for you.

Complementary stretches
A02, A07.

A05: NECK EXTENSION STRETCH

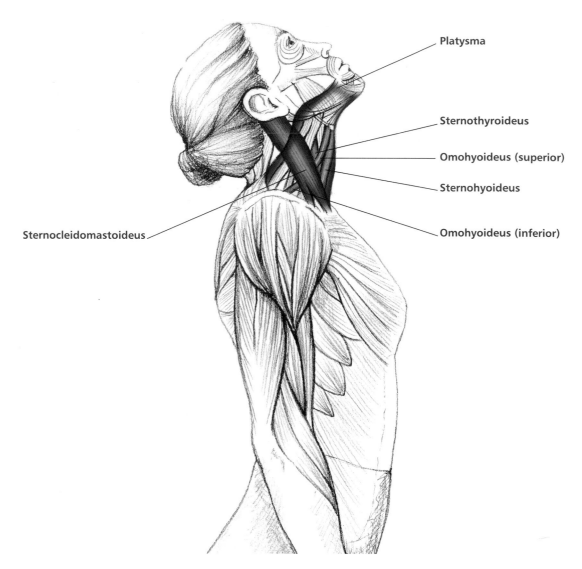

Platysma

Sternothyroideus

Omohyoideus (superior)

Sternohyoideus

Omohyoideus (inferior)

Sternocleidomastoideus

Technique
Stand upright and lift your head, looking upwards as if trying to point up with your chin. Relax your shoulders and keep your hands by your side.

Muscles being stretched
Primary muscles: Platysma. Sternocleidomastoideus.
Secondary muscles: Omohyoideus. Sternohyoideus. Sternothyroideus.

Sports that benefit from this stretch
Boxing. American football (gridiron). Rugby. Cycling. Swimming. Wrestling.

Sports injury where stretch may be useful
Neck muscle strain. Whiplash (neck sprain). Cervical nerve stretch syndrome. Wryneck (acute torticollis).

Additional information for performing this stretch correctly
Keep your mouth closed and your teeth together when doing this stretch.

Complementary stretch
C02.

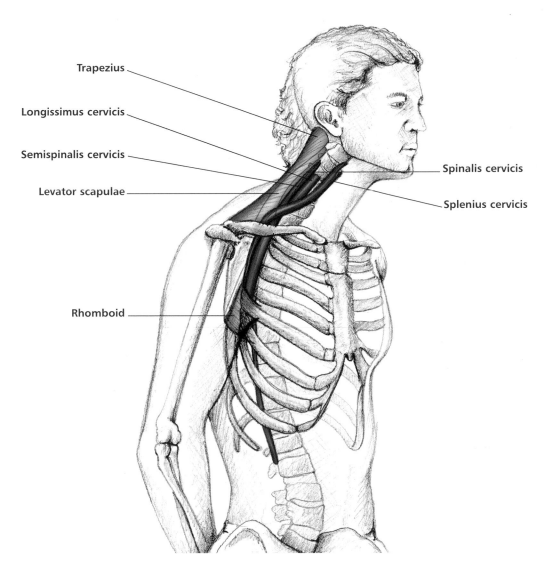

Trapezius

Longissimus cervicis

Semispinalis cervicis

Levator scapulae

Rhomboid

Spinalis cervicis

Splenius cervicis

Technique
Keep your head up then push your head forward by sticking your chin out.

Muscles being stretched
Primary muscles: Semispinalis cervicis. Spinalis cervicis. Longissimus cervicis. Splenius cervicis. Secondary muscles: Levator scapulae. Trapezius. Rhomboids.

Sports that benefit from this stretch
Boxing. American football (gridiron). Rugby. Cycling. Swimming. Wrestling.

Sports injury where stretch may be useful
Neck muscle strain. Whiplash (neck sprain). Cervical nerve stretch syndrome. Wryneck (acute torticollis).

Additional information for performing this stretch correctly
Keep your head up. Do not let your chin fall towards the ground.

Complementary stretch
A03.

A07: SITTING NECK FLEXION STRETCH

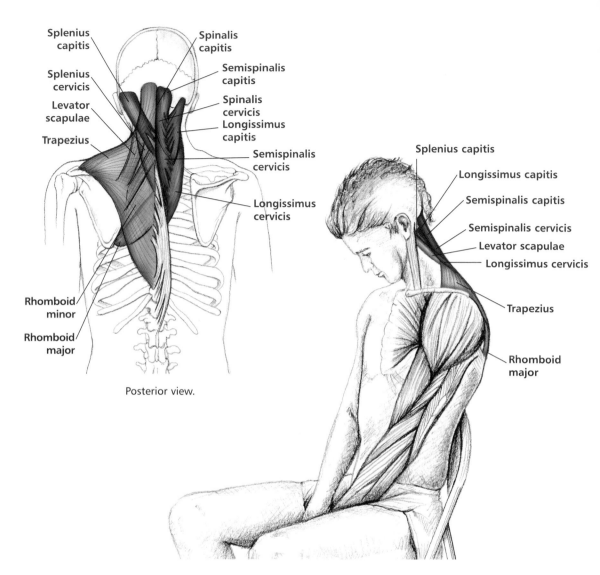

Posterior view.

Technique
While sitting on a chair, cross your arms over and hang on to the chair between your legs. Let your head fall forward and then lean backwards.

Muscles being stretched
Primary muscles: Semispinalis capitis and cervicis. Spinalis capitis and cervicis. Longissimus capitis and cervicis. Splenius capitis and cervicis. Secondary muscles: Levator scapulae. Trapezius. Rhomboids.

Sports that benefit from this stretch
Archery. Boxing. American football (gridiron). Rugby. Cycling. Golf. Swimming. Wrestling.

Sports injury where stretch may be useful
Neck muscle strain. Whiplash (neck sprain). Cervical nerve stretch syndrome. Wryneck (acute torticollis).

Common problems and more information for performing this stretch correctly
Some people are more flexible in the upper back and neck than others. Do not overstretch by forcing your head down: instead, relax and let the weight of your head do the stretching for you.

Complementary stretches
A03, A11.

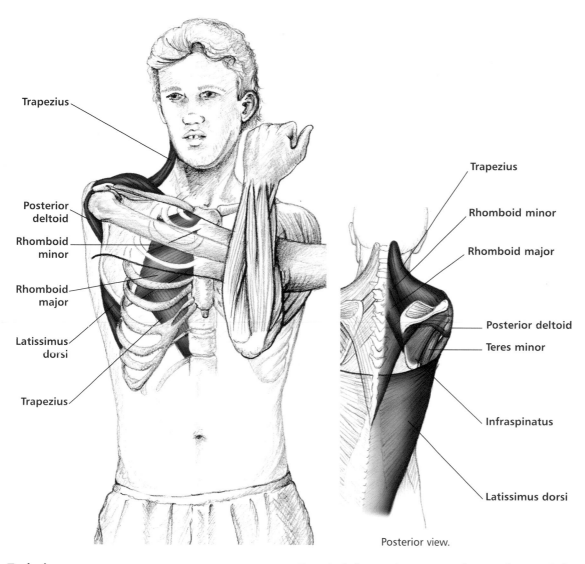

Trapezius

Posterior deltoid

Rhomboid minor

Rhomboid major

Latissimus dorsi

Trapezius

Trapezius

Rhomboid minor

Rhomboid major

Posterior deltoid

Teres minor

Infraspinatus

Latissimus dorsi

Posterior view.

Technique
Stand upright and place one arm across your body. Keep your arm parallel to the ground and pull your elbow towards your opposite shoulder.

Muscles being stretched
Primary muscles: Trapezius. Rhomboids. Latissimus dorsi. Posterior deltoid. Secondary muscles: Infraspinatus. Teres minor.

Sports that benefit from this stretch
Archery. Cricket. Baseball. Softball. Boxing. Golf. Tennis. Badminton. Squash. Rowing. Canoeing. Kayaking. Swimming. Athletics throwing field events.

Sports injury where stretch may be useful
Dislocation. Subluxation. Acromioclavicular separation. Sternoclavicular separation. Impingement syndrome. Rotator cuff tendonitis. Shoulder bursitis. Frozen shoulder (adhesive capsulitis).

Additional information for performing this stretch correctly
Keep your arm straight and parallel to the ground.

Complementary stretch
A09.

A09: BENT ARM SHOULDER STRETCH

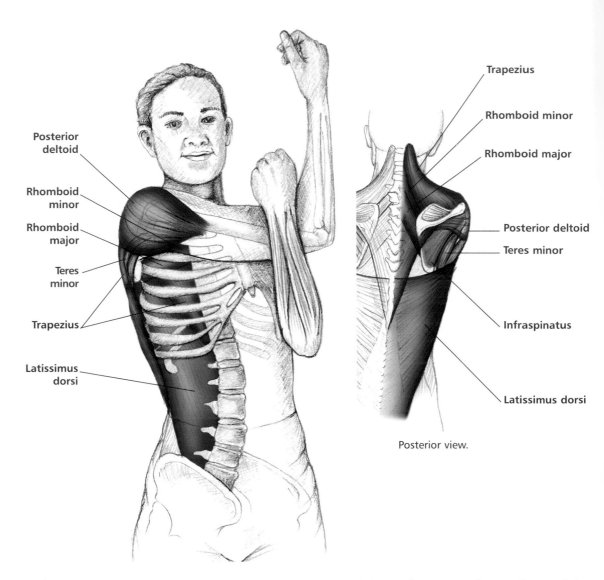

Posterior deltoid

Rhomboid minor

Rhomboid major

Teres minor

Trapezius

Latissimus dorsi

Trapezius

Rhomboid minor

Rhomboid major

Posterior deltoid

Teres minor

Infraspinatus

Latissimus dorsi

Posterior view.

Technique
Stand upright and place one arm across your body. Bend your arm at 90 degrees and pull your elbow towards your opposite shoulder.

Muscles being stretched
Primary muscles: Trapezius. Rhomboids. Latissimus dorsi. Posterior deltoid. Secondary muscles: Infraspinatus. Teres minor.

Sports that benefit from this stretch
Archery. Cricket. Baseball. Softball. Boxing. Golf. Tennis. Badminton. Squash. Rowing. Canoeing. Kayaking. Swimming. Athletics throwing field events.

Sports injury where stretch may be useful
Dislocation. Subluxation. Acromioclavicular separation. Sternoclavicular separation. Impingement syndrome. Rotator cuff tendonitis. Shoulder bursitis. Frozen shoulder (adhesive capsulitis).

Additional information for performing this stretch correctly
Keep your upper arm parallel to the ground.

Complementary stretch
A08.

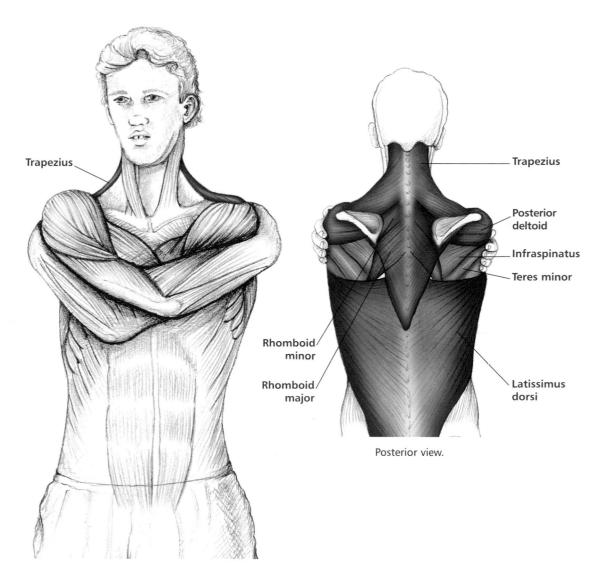

Posterior view.

Technique
Stand upright and wrap your arms around your shoulders as if hugging yourself. Pull your shoulders back.

Muscles being stretched
Primary muscles: Trapezius. Rhomboids. Latissimus dorsi. Posterior deltoid. Secondary muscles: Infraspinatus. Teres minor.

Sports that benefit from this stretch
Archery. Cricket. Baseball. Softball. Boxing. Golf. Tennis. Badminton. Squash. Rowing. Canoeing. Kayaking. Swimming. Athletics throwing field events.

Sports injury where stretch may be useful
Dislocation. Subluxation. Acromioclavicular separation. Sternoclavicular separation. Impingement syndrome. Rotator cuff tendonitis. Shoulder bursitis. Frozen shoulder (adhesive capsulitis).

Common problems and more information for performing this stretch correctly
Do not pull too quickly on your shoulders. Ease into the stretch by slowly pulling your shoulders back.

Complementary stretch
A11.

A11: CROSS OVER SHOULDER STRETCH

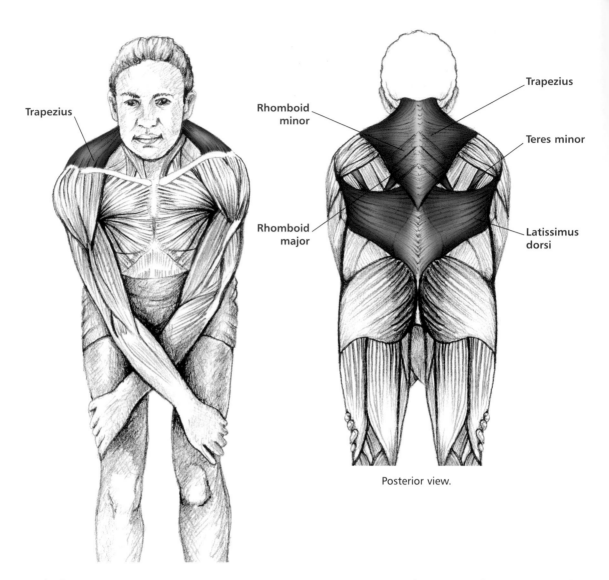

Trapezius

Rhomboid minor

Rhomboid major

Trapezius

Teres minor

Latissimus dorsi

Posterior view.

Technique
Stand with your knees bent. Cross your arms over and grab the back of your knees. Then start to rise upwards until you feel tension in your upper back and shoulders.

Muscles being stretched
Primary muscles: Trapezius. Rhomboids. Latissimus dorsi.
Secondary muscle: Teres minor.

Sports that benefit from this stretch
Archery. Cricket. Baseball. Softball. Boxing. Golf. Tennis. Badminton. Squash. Rowing. Canoeing. Kayaking. Swimming. Athletics throwing field events.

Sports injury where stretch may be useful
Dislocation. Subluxation. Acromioclavicular separation. Sternoclavicular separation. Impingement syndrome. Rotator cuff tendonitis. Shoulder bursitis. Frozen shoulder (adhesive capsulitis).

Common problems and more information for performing this stretch correctly
Keep your shoulders level to the ground and avoid twisting or turning to one side.

Complementary stretch
A07.

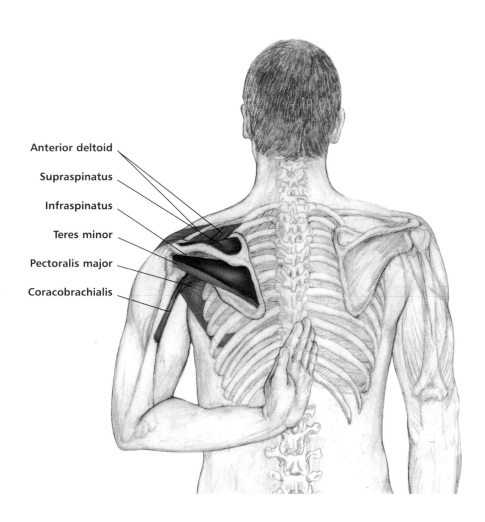

Anterior deltoid

Supraspinatus

Infraspinatus

Teres minor

Pectoralis major

Coracobrachialis

Technique
Place one hand behind your back and then reach up between your shoulder-blades.

Muscles being stretched
Primary muscles: Supraspinatus. Infraspinatus.
Secondary muscles: Pectoralis major. Teres minor. Anterior deltoid. Coracobrachialis.

Sports that benefit from this stretch
Martial arts. Tennis. Badminton. Squash. Rowing. Canoeing. Kayaking. Swimming. Cricket. Baseball. Field events. Wrestling.

Sports injury where stretch may be useful
Dislocation. Subluxation. Acromioclavicular separation. Sternoclavicular separation. Impingement syndrome. Rotator cuff tendonitis. Shoulder bursitis. Frozen shoulder (adhesive capsulitis).

Common problems and more information for performing this stretch correctly
Many people are very tight in the rotator muscles of the shoulder. Perform this stretch very slowly to start with and use extreme caution at all times.

Complementary stretches
A13, A15.

A13: ELBOW-OUT ROTATOR STRETCH

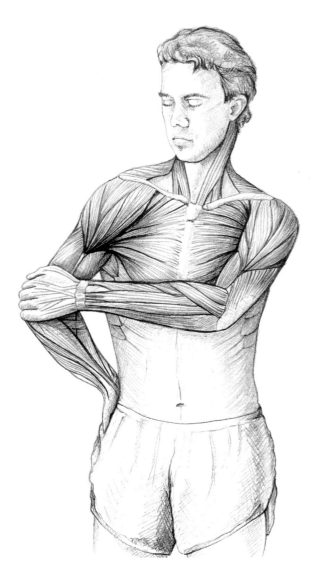

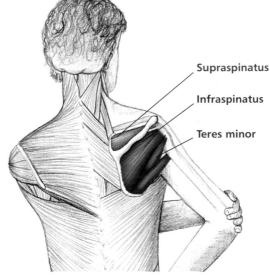

Supraspinatus

Infraspinatus

Teres minor

Technique
Stand with your hand behind the middle of your back and your elbow pointing out. Reach over with your other hand and gently pull your elbow forward.

Muscles being stretched
Primary muscles: Infraspinatus. Teres minor. Secondary muscle: Supraspinatus.

Sports that benefit from this stretch
Martial arts. Tennis. Badminton. Squash. Rowing. Canoeing. Kayaking. Swimming. Cricket. Baseball. Athletics throwing field events. Wrestling.

Sports injury where stretch may be useful
Dislocation. Subluxation. Acromioclavicular separation. Sternoclavicular separation. Impingement syndrome. Rotator cuff tendonitis. Shoulder bursitis. Frozen shoulder (adhesive capsulitis).

Common problems and additional information for performing this stretch correctly
Many people are very tight in the rotator cuff muscles of the shoulder. Perform this stretch very slowly to start with and use extreme caution at all times.

Complementary stretch
A15.

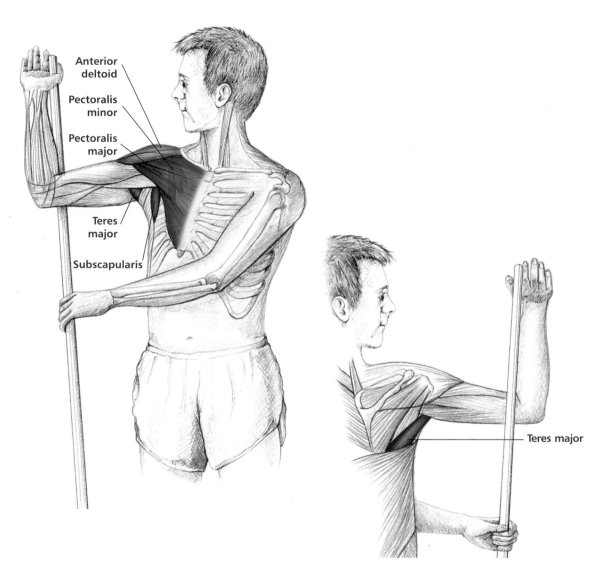

Anterior deltoid

Pectoralis minor

Pectoralis major

Teres major

Subscapularis

Teres major

Technique
Stand with your arm out and your forearm pointing upwards at 90 degrees. Place a broomstick in your hand and behind your elbow. With your other hand pull the bottom of the broomstick forward.

Muscles being stretched
Primary muscles: Pectoralis major.
Subscapularis. Teres major.
Secondary muscle: Pectoralis minor. Anterior deltoid.

Sports that benefit from this stretch
Martial arts. Tennis. Badminton. Squash. Rowing. Canoeing. Kayaking. Swimming. Cricket. Baseball. Athletics throwing field events. Wrestling.

Sports injury where stretch may be useful
Dislocation. Subluxation. Acromioclavicular separation. Sternoclavicular separation. Impingement syndrome. Rotator cuff tendonitis. Shoulder bursitis. Frozen shoulder (adhesive capsulitis).

Common problems and additional information for performing this stretch correctly
Many people are very tight in the rotator cuff muscles of the shoulder. Perform this stretch very slowly to start with and use extreme caution at all times.

Complementary stretch
A15.

A15: ARM-DOWN ROTATOR STRETCH

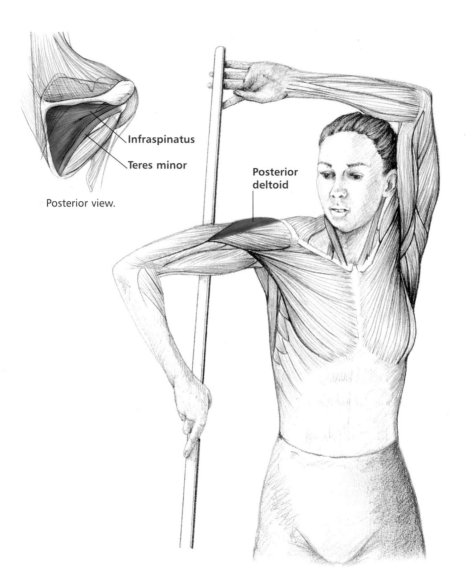

Infraspinatus

Teres minor

Posterior view.

Posterior deltoid

Technique
Stand with your arm out and your forearm pointing downwards at 90 degrees. Place a broomstick in your hand and behind your elbow. With your other hand pull the top of the broomstick forward.

Muscles being stretched
Primary muscle: Infraspinatus. Posterior deltoid.
Secondary muscle: Teres minor.

Sports that benefit from this stretch
Martial arts. Tennis. Badminton. Squash. Rowing. Canoeing. Kayaking. Swimming. Cricket. Baseball. Athletics throwing field events. Wrestling.

Sports injury where stretch may be useful
Dislocation. Subluxation. Acromioclavicular separation. Sternoclavicular separation. Impingement syndrome. Rotator cuff tendonitis. Shoulder bursitis. Frozen shoulder (adhesive capsulitis).

Common problems and additional information for performing this stretch correctly
Many people are very tight in the rotator cuff muscles of the shoulder. Perform this stretch very slowly to start with and use extreme caution at all times.

Complementary stretch
A13.

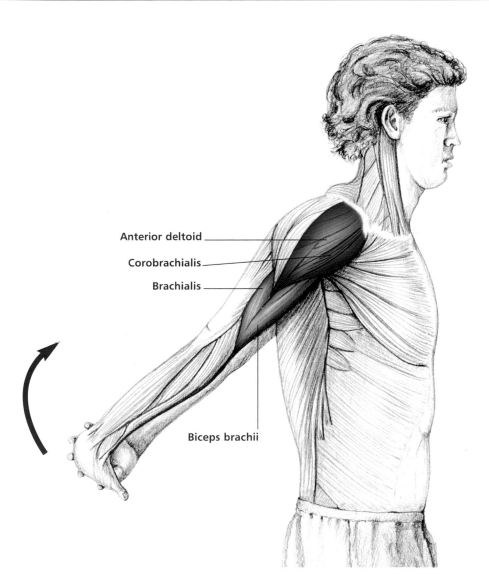

Anterior deltoid

Corobrachialis

Brachialis

Biceps brachii

Technique
Stand upright and clasp your hands together behind your back. Slowly lift your hands upward.

Muscles being stretched
Primary muscle: Anterior deltoid.
Secondary muscles. Biceps brachii. Brachialis. Coracobrachialis.

Sports that benefit from this stretch
Basketball. Netball. Hiking. Backpacking. Mountaineering. Orienteering. Tennis. Badminton. Squash. Rowing. Canoeing. Kayaking. Swimming. Cricket. Baseball. Athletics throwing field events.

Sports injury where stretch may be useful
Dislocation. Subluxation. Acromioclavicular separation. Sternoclavicular separation. Impingement syndrome. Rotator cuff tendonitis. Shoulder bursitis. Frozen shoulder (adhesive capsulitis). Chest strain. Pectoral muscle insertion inflammation.

Additional information for performing this stretch correctly
Do not lean forward while lifting your hands upward.

Complementary stretch
B06.

A17: ASSISTED REVERSE SHOULDER STRETCH

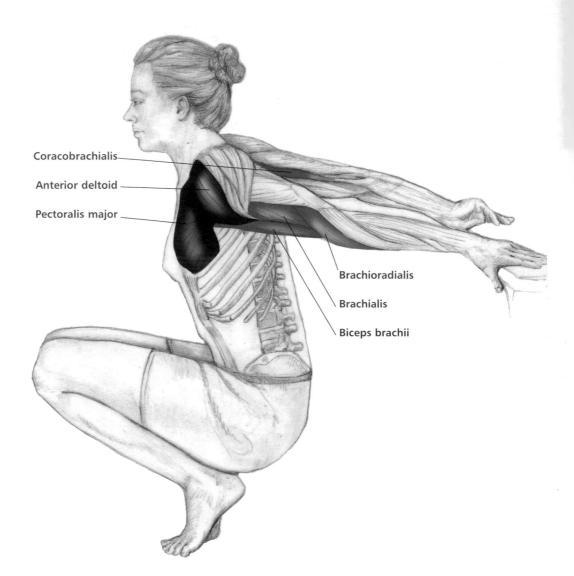

Coracobrachialis

Anterior deltoid

Pectoralis major

Brachioradialis

Brachialis

Biceps brachii

Technique
Stand upright with your back towards a table or bench and place your hands on the edge of the table or bench. Keep your arms straight and slowly lower your entire body.

Muscles being stretched
Primary muscles: Anterior deltoid. Pectoralis major.
Secondary muscles: Biceps brachii. Brachialis. Brachioradialis. Coracobrachialis.

Sports that benefit from this stretch
Basketball. Netball. Hiking. Backpacking. Mountaineering. Orienteering. Tennis. Badminton. Squash. Rowing. Canoeing. Kayaking. Swimming. Cricket. Baseball. Field events.

Sports injury where stretch may be useful
Dislocation. Subluxation. Acromioclavicular separation. Sternoclavicular separation. Impingement syndrome. Rotator cuff tendonitis. Shoulder bursitis. Frozen shoulder (adhesive capsulitis). Chest strain. Pectoral muscle insertion inflammation.

Common problems and more information for performing this stretch correctly
Look forward and keep your body upright.

Complementary stretches
B03, B05.

4 Arms and Chest

Mobility of the upper limb is mainly dependent on three joints: the sternoclavicular, acromioclavicular, and shoulder joints. Muscles in this area can be categorised according to: 1) muscles that run between the trunk and the scapula, which act upon the shoulder girdle and not on the shoulder joint, i.e., **trapezius**, **levator scapulae**, **rhomboids**, **serratus anterior**, **pectoralis minor**, and **subclavius**; 2) muscles that run between the trunk and the humerus, which act upon the shoulder joint and the shoulder girdle: i.e., **latissimus dorsi** and **pectoralis major**; 3) muscles that run between the scapula and humerus, which act exclusively upon the shoulder joint, i.e., **deltoideus**, **supraspinatus**, **infraspinatus**, **teres minor**, **subscapularis**, **teres major**, and **coracobrachialis**.

Muscles of the arm comprise those that originate from the scapula and/or the humerus, and insert into the radius and/or ulna, so that they act upon the elbow joint. These are: **biceps brachii**; **brachialis**; **triceps brachii**; and **anconeus**. **Coracobrachialis**, although acting upon the shoulder joint, is also included because of its proximity to the other muscles of this group. **Biceps brachii** operates over three joints, and has two tendinous heads at its origin and two tendinous insertions. Occasionally it has a third head, originating at the insertion of coracobrachialis. The short head forms part of the lateral wall of the axilla, along with coracobrachialis and the humerus. **Brachialis** lies posterior to biceps brachii and is the main flexor of the elbow joint. **Triceps brachii** originates from three heads and is the only muscle on the back of the arm.

The anterior forearm contains three functional muscle groups: the pronators of the forearm; the wrist flexors; and the long flexors of the fingers and thumb. They are arranged in three layers: the superficial layer comprises four muscles: **pronator teres**; **flexor carpi radialis**; **palmaris longus**; and **flexor carpi ulnaris**. The middle layer contains only the **flexor digitorum superficialis**. The deepest layer consists of: **flexor digitorum profundus**; **flexor pollicis longus**; and **pronator quadratus**. On the back of the forearm there are two muscle groups. The superficial group contains, from the radial to ulnar side: **brachioradialis**; **extensor carpi radialis longus**; **extensor carpi radialis brevis**; **extensor digitorum**; **extensor digiti minimi**; and **extensor carpi ulnaris**. The muscle belly of brachioradialis is prominent when working against resistance. The deep group contains: **supinator**; **abductor pollicis longus**; **extensor pollicis brevis**; **extensor pollicis longus**; and **extensor indicis**.

The muscle groupings in the hand are: 1) the "intrinsic" muscles, consisting of the **interossei**, located within the intermetacarpal spaces to act on the four fingers and thumb, and the **lumbricals**, which arise from the tendons of flexor digitorum profundus in the palm and act on the four fingers; 2) the muscles of the hypothenar eminence; 3) the muscles of the thenar eminence; 4) **adductor pollicis**.

Sports that benefit from these arm and chest stretches include: archery; basketball and netball; batting sports like cricket, baseball, and softball; hiking, backpacking, mountaineering, and orienteering; ice hockey and field hockey; martial arts; racquet sports like tennis, badminton, and squash; rowing, canoeing, and kayaking; swimming; throwing sports like cricket, baseball, and field events; volleyball; wrestling.

B01: ABOVE HEAD CHEST STRETCH

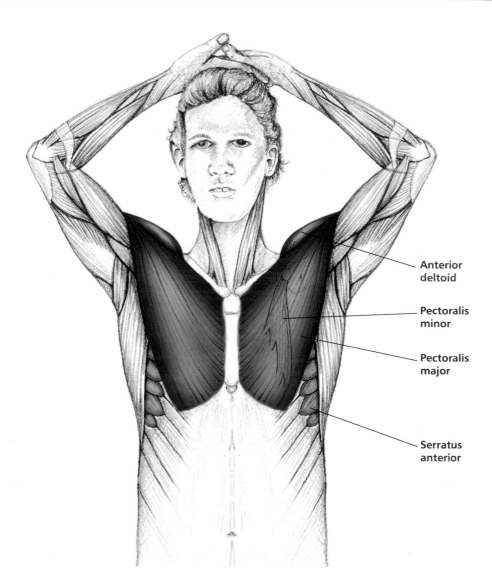

Anterior deltoid

Pectoralis minor

Pectoralis major

Serratus anterior

Technique
Stand upright and interlock your fingers. Bend your arms and place them above your head while forcing your elbows and hands backwards.

Muscles being stretched
Primary muscles: Pectoralis major and minor. Anterior deltoid.
Secondary muscle: Serratus anterior.

Sports that benefit from this stretch
Basketball. Netball. Hiking. Backpacking. Mountaineering. Orienteering. Tennis. Badminton. Squash. Rowing. Canoeing. Kayaking. Swimming. Cricket. Baseball. Athletics throwing field events.

Sports injury where stretch may be useful
Impingement syndrome. Rotator cuff tendonitis. Shoulder bursitis. Frozen shoulder (adhesive capsulitis). Chest strain. Pectoral muscle insertion inflammation.

Additional information for performing this stretch correctly
Vary the height of your hands. Lower your hands behind your head to place an emphasis on the *anterior deltoid* and raise your hands above your head to emphasize the *pectoral* muscles.

Complementary stretch
B07.

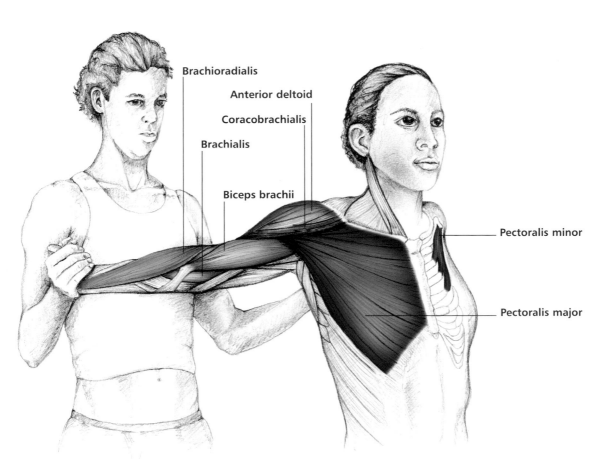

Brachioradialis

Anterior deltoid

Coracobrachialis

Brachialis

Biceps brachii

Pectoralis minor

Pectoralis major

Technique

Extend both of your arms parallel to the ground. Have a partner hold on to your hands and slowly pull your arms backwards.

Muscles being stretched

Primary muscles: Pectoralis major and minor. Anterior deltoid.
Secondary muscles: Biceps brachii. Brachialis. Brachioradialis. Coracobrachialis.

Sports that benefit from this stretch

Basketball. Netball. Hiking. Backpacking. Mountaineering. Orienteering. Tennis. Badminton. Squash. Rowing. Canoeing. Kayaking. Swimming. Cricket. Baseball. Athletics throwing field events.

Sports injury where stretch may be useful

Dislocation. Subluxation. Acromioclavicular separation. Sternoclavicular separation. Impingement syndrome. Rotator cuff tendonitis. Shoulder bursitis. Frozen shoulder (adhesive capsulitis). Biceps tendon rupture. Bicepital tendonitis. Biceps strain. Chest strain. Pectoral muscle insertion inflammation.

Additional information for performing this stretch correctly

Keep your arms parallel to the ground and your palms facing outward.

Complementary stretch

B04.

B03: SEATED PARTNER ASSISTED CHEST STRETCH

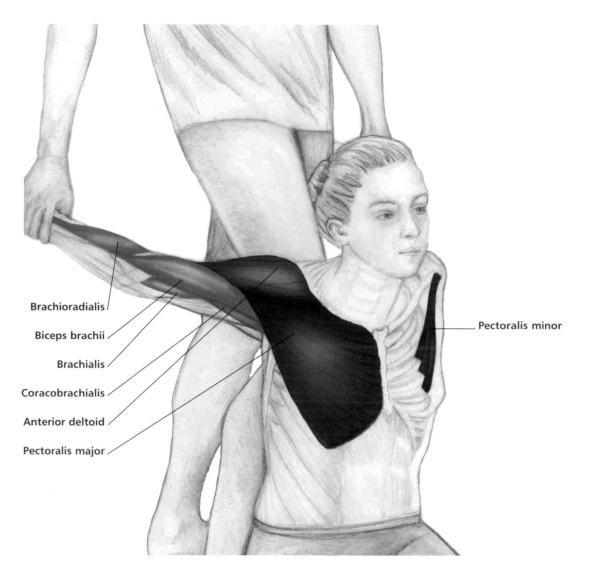

Brachioradialis

Biceps brachii

Brachialis

Coracobrachialis

Anterior deltoid

Pectoralis major

Pectoralis minor

Technique
Sit on the ground and have a partner stand behind you. Reach behind with both arms and have the partner further extend your arms.

Muscles being stretched
Primary muscles: Pectoralis major and minor. Anterior deltoid.
Secondary muscles: Biceps brachii. Brachialis. Brachioradialis. Coracobrachialis.

Sports that benefit from this stretch
Basketball. Netball. Hiking. Backpacking. Mountaineering. Orienteering. Tennis. Badminton. Squash. Rowing. Canoeing. Kayaking. Swimming. Cricket. Baseball. Field events.

Sports injury where stretch may be useful
Dislocation. Subluxation. Acromioclavicular separation. Sternoclavicular separation. Impingement syndrome. Rotator cuff tendonitis. Shoulder bursitis. Frozen shoulder (adhesive capsulitis). Biceps tendon rupture. Bicepital tendonitis. Biceps strain. Chest strain. Pectoral muscle insertion inflammation.

Common problems and more information for performing this stretch correctly
Keep your palms facing outward and your arms slightly above parallel to the ground.

Complementary stretches
B01, B05.

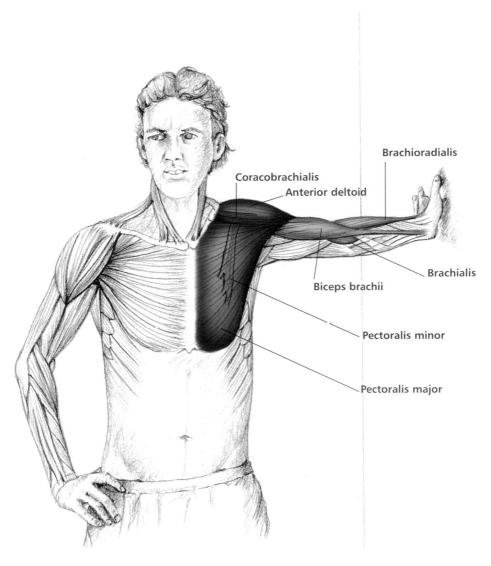

Coracobrachialis

Brachioradialis

Anterior deltoid

Brachialis

Biceps brachii

Pectoralis minor

Pectoralis major

Technique
Stand with your arm extended to the rear and parallel to the ground. Hold on to an immovable object and then turn your shoulders and body away from your outstretched arm.

Muscles being stretched
Primary muscles: Pectoralis major and minor. Anterior deltoid.
Secondary muscles: Biceps brachii. Brachialis. Brachioradialis. Coracobrachialis.

Sports that benefit from this stretch
Basketball. Netball. Hiking. Backpacking. Mountaineering. Orienteering. Tennis. Badminton. Squash. Rowing. Canoeing. Kayaking. Swimming. Cricket. Baseball. Athletics throwing field events.

Sports injury where stretch may be useful
Dislocation. Subluxation. Acromioclavicular separation. Sternoclavicular separation. Impingement syndrome. Rotator cuff tendonitis. Shoulder bursitis. Frozen shoulder (adhesive capsulitis). Biceps tendon rupture. Bicepital tendonitis. Biceps strain. Chest strain. Pectoral muscle insertion inflammation.

Additional information for performing this stretch correctly
Keep your arm parallel to the ground and your fingers pointing backwards.

Complementary stretch
B02.

B05: BENT ARM CHEST STRETCH

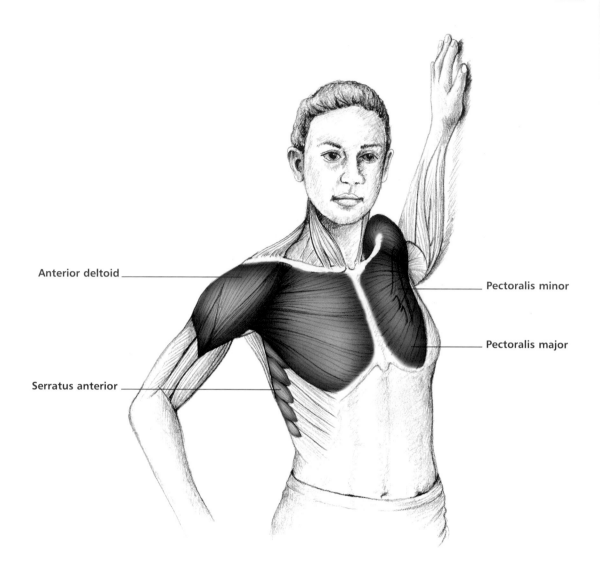

Anterior deltoid

Serratus anterior

Pectoralis minor

Pectoralis major

Technique
Stand with your arm extended and your forearm at right angles to the ground. Rest your forearm against an immovable object and then turn your shoulders and body away from your extended arm.

Muscles being stretched
Primary muscles: Pectoralis major and minor. Anterior deltoid.
Secondary muscle: Serratus anterior.

Sports that benefit from this stretch
Basketball. Netball. Hiking. Backpacking. Mountaineering. Orienteering. Tennis. Badminton. Squash. Rowing. Canoeing. Kayaking. Swimming. Cricket. Baseball. Athletics throwing field events.

Sports injury where stretch may be useful
Dislocation. Subluxation. Acromioclavicular separation. Sternoclavicular separation. Impingement syndrome. Rotator cuff tendonitis. Shoulder bursitis. Frozen shoulder (adhesive capsulitis). Chest strain. Pectoral muscle insertion inflammation.

Additional information for performing this stretch correctly
Keep your upper arm parallel to the ground.

Complementary stretch
B04.

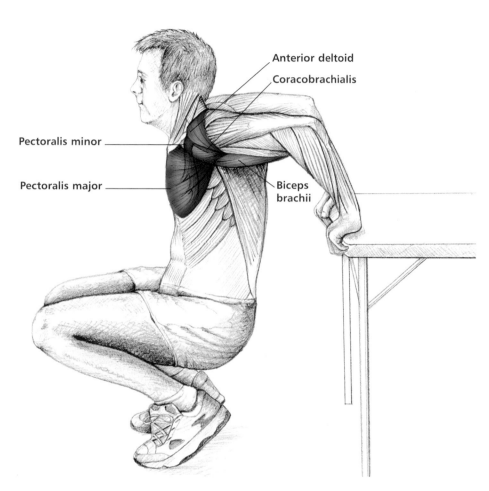

Anterior deltoid

Coracobrachialis

Pectoralis minor

Pectoralis major

Biceps brachii

Technique
Stand upright with your back towards a table or bench and place your hands on the edge of the table or bench. Slowly lower your entire body.

Muscles being stretched
Primary muscles: Anterior deltoid. Pectoralis major and minor.
Secondary muscles: Biceps brachii. Coracobrachialis.

Sports that benefit from this stretch
Archery. Cricket. Baseball. Softball. Boxing. Golf. Tennis. Badminton. Squash. Rowing. Canoeing. Kayaking. Swimming. Athletics throwing field events.

Sports injury where stretch may be useful
Dislocation. Subluxation. Acromioclavicular separation. Sternoclavicular separation. Impingement syndrome. Rotator cuff tendonitis. Shoulder bursitis. Frozen shoulder (adhesive capsulitis). Biceps tendon rupture. Bicepital tendonitis. Biceps strain. Chest strain. Pectoral muscle insertion inflammation.

Common problems and additional information for performing this stretch correctly
Use your legs to control the lowering of your body. Do not lower your body too quickly.

Complementary stretch
A16.

B07: BENT-OVER CHEST STRETCH

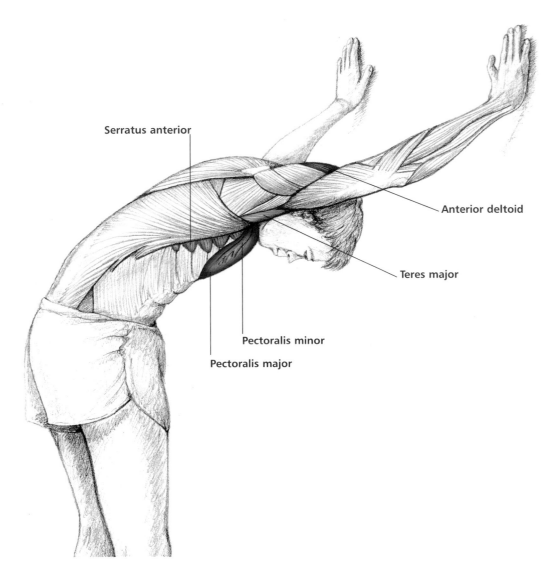

Serratus anterior

Anterior deltoid

Teres major

Pectoralis minor

Pectoralis major

Technique
Face a wall and place both hands on the wall just above your head. Slowly lower your shoulders as if moving your chin towards the ground.

Muscles being stretched
Primary muscles: Pectoralis major and minor. Anterior deltoid.
Secondary muscles: Serratus anterior. Teres major.

Sports that benefit from this stretch
Basketball. Netball. Hiking. Backpacking. Mountaineering. Orienteering. Tennis. Badminton. Squash. Rowing. Canoeing. Kayaking. Swimming. Cricket. Baseball. Athletics throwing field events.

Sports injury where stretch may be useful
Dislocation. Subluxation. Acromioclavicular separation. Sternoclavicular separation. Impingement syndrome. Rotator cuff tendonitis. Shoulder bursitis. Frozen shoulder (adhesive capsulitis). Chest strain. Pectoral muscle insertion inflammation.

Additional information for performing this stretch correctly
Keep your arms straight and your fingers pointing straight upwards.

Complementary stretch
B01.

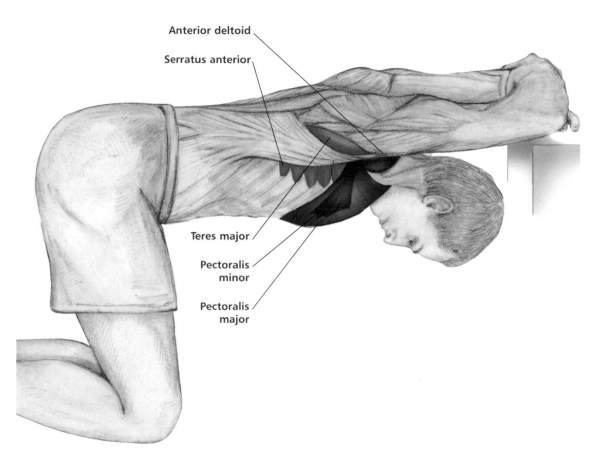

Anterior deltoid

Serratus anterior

Teres major

Pectoralis minor

Pectoralis major

Technique
Kneel on the floor in front of a chair or table and interlock your forearms above your head. Place your arms on the object and lower your upper body toward the ground.

Muscles being stretched
Primary muscles: Pectoralis major and minor. Anterior deltoid.
Secondary muscles: Serratus anterior. Teres major.

Sports that benefit from this stretch
Basketball. Netball. Hiking. Backpacking. Mountaineering. Orienteering. Tennis. Badminton. Squash. Rowing. Canoeing. Kayaking. Swimming. Cricket. Baseball. Field events.

Sports injury where stretch may be useful
Impingement syndrome. Rotator cuff tendonitis. Shoulder bursitis. Frozen shoulder (adhesive capsulitis). Chest strain. Pectoral muscle insertion inflammation.

Common problems and more information for performing this stretch correctly
Keep your elbows bent and vary the width of your arms for a slightly different stretch.

Complementary stretches
B01, B07.

B09: REACHING-DOWN TRICEPS STRETCH

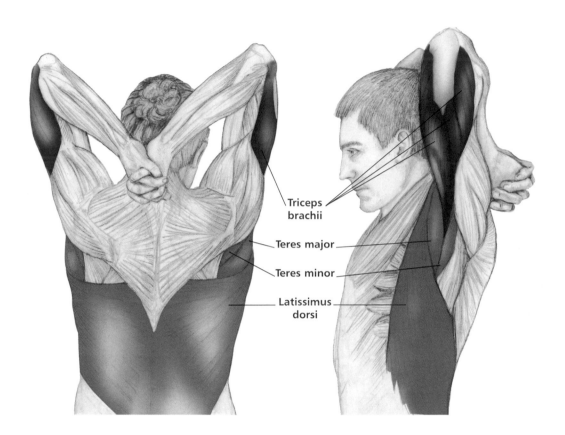

Triceps brachii

Teres major

Teres minor

Latissimus dorsi

Technique
Reach behind your head with both hands and your elbows pointing upwards. Then reach down your back with your hands.

Muscles being stretched
Primary muscle. Triceps brachii.
Secondary muscles: Latissimus dorsi. Teres major and minor.

Sports that benefit from this stretch
Basketball. Netball. Tennis. Badminton. Squash. Rowing. Canoeing. Kayaking. Swimming. Cricket. Baseball. Field events. Volleyball.

Sports injury where stretch may be useful
Elbow sprain. Elbow dislocation. Elbow bursitis. Triceps tendon rupture.

Common problems and more information for performing this stretch correctly
Do not perform for an extended period of time, as circulation is restricted in the shoulder during this stretch.

Complementary stretches
A14, B08.

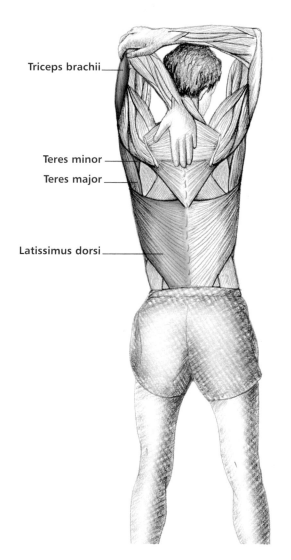

Triceps brachii

Teres minor

Teres major

Latissimus dorsi

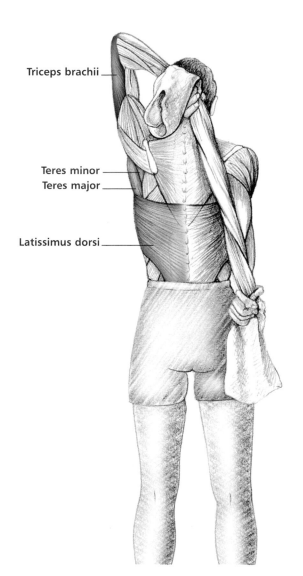

Triceps brachii

Teres minor

Teres major

Latissimus dorsi

Technique
Stand with your hand behind your neck and your elbow pointing upwards. Then use your other hand (or a rope or towel) to pull your elbow down.

Muscles being stretched
Primary muscle: Triceps brachii.
Secondary muscles: Latissimus dorsi. Teres major and minor.

Sports that benefit from this stretch
Basketball. Netball. Tennis. Badminton. Squash. Rowing. Canoeing. Kayaking. Swimming. Cricket. Baseball. Athletics throwing field events. Volleyball.

Sports injury where stretch may be useful
Elbow sprain. Elbow dislocation. Elbow bursitis. Triceps tendon rupture.

Common problems and additional information for performing this stretch correctly
Do not perform this stretch for an extended period of time, as the blood circulation is restricted in the shoulder.

Complementary stretch
D03.

B11: KNEELING FOREARM STRETCH

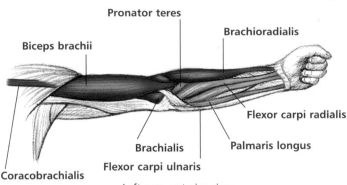

Pronator teres

Biceps brachii

Brachioradialis

Flexor carpi radialis

Coracobrachialis

Brachialis

Flexor carpi ulnaris

Palmaris longus

Left arm, anterior view.

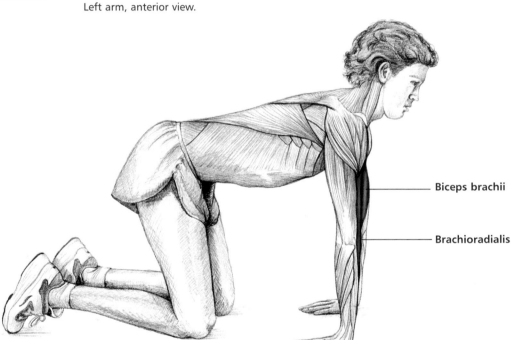

Biceps brachii

Brachioradialis

Technique
While crouching on your knees with your forearms facing forward and hands pointing backwards, slowly move rearward.

Muscles being stretched
Primary muscles: Biceps brachii. Brachialis. Brachioradialis. Coracobrachialis.
Secondary muscles: Pronator teres. Flexor carpi radialis. Flexor carpi ulnaris. Palmaris longus.

Sports that benefit from this stretch
Basketball. Netball. Cricket. Baseball. Softball. Ice hockey. Field hockey. Martial arts. Tennis. Badminton. Squash. Rowing. Canoeing. Kayaking. Swimming. Athletics throwing field events. Volleyball. Wrestling.

Sports injury where stretch may be useful
Biceps tendon rupture. Bicipital tendonitis. Biceps strain. Elbow strain. Elbow dislocation. Elbow bursitis. Tennis elbow. Golfer's elbow. Thrower's elbow.

Common problems and more information for performing this stretch correctly
Depending on where your muscles are most tight, you may feel this stretch more in your forearms or more in your upper arms. To make this stretch easier, move your hands towards your knees.

Complementary stretch
B12.

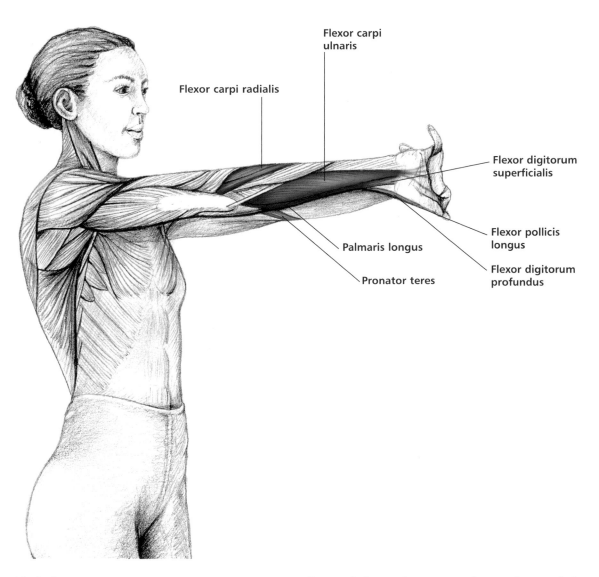

Flexor carpi ulnaris

Flexor carpi radialis

Flexor digitorum superficialis

Flexor pollicis longus

Flexor digitorum profundus

Palmaris longus

Pronator teres

Technique
Interlock your fingers in front of your chest and then straighten your arms and turn the palms of your hands outwards.

Muscles being stretched
Primary muscles: Pronator teres. Flexor carpi radialis. Flexor carpi ulnaris. Palmaris longus. Secondary muscles: Flexor digitorum superficialis. Flexor digitorum profundus. Flexor pollicis longus.

Sports that benefit from this stretch
Basketball. Netball. Cricket. Baseball. Softball. Ice hockey. Field hockey. Martial arts. Tennis. Badminton. Squash. Rowing. Canoeing. Kayaking. Swimming. Athletics throwing field events. Volleyball. Wrestling.

Sports injury where stretch may be useful
Tennis elbow. Golfer's elbow. Thrower's elbow. Wrist sprain. Wrist dislocation. Wrist tendonitis. Carpal tunnel syndrome. Ulnar tunnel syndrome.

Common problems and more information for performing this stretch correctly
The forearms, wrists, and fingers comprise a multitude of small muscles, tendons, and ligaments. Do not overstretch this area by applying too much force too quickly.

Complementary stretch
B13.

B13: FINGERS-DOWN FOREARM STRETCH

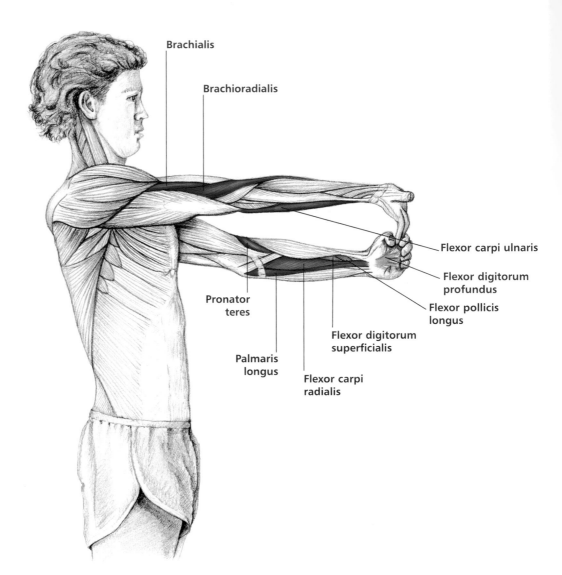

Brachialis

Brachioradialis

Flexor carpi ulnaris

Flexor digitorum profundus

Flexor pollicis longus

Pronator teres

Flexor digitorum superficialis

Palmaris longus

Flexor carpi radialis

Technique
Hold onto your fingers and turn your palms outwards. Straighten your arm and then pull your fingers back using your other hand.

Muscles being stretched
Primary muscles: Brachialis. Brachioradialis. Pronator teres. Flexor carpi radialis. Flexor carpi ulnaris. Palmaris longus.
Secondary muscles: Flexor digitorum superficialis. Flexor digitorum profundus. Flexor pollicis longus.

Sports that benefit from this stretch
Basketball. Netball. Cricket. Baseball. Softball. Ice hockey. Field hockey. Martial arts. Tennis. Badminton. Squash. Rowing. Canoeing. Kayaking. Swimming. Athletics throwing field events. Volleyball. Wrestling.

Sports injury where stretch may be useful
Tennis elbow. Golfer's elbow. Thrower's elbow. Wrist sprain. Wrist dislocation. Wrist tendonitis. Carpal tunnel syndrome. Ulnar tunnel syndrome.

Common problems and more information for performing this stretch correctly
The forearms, wrists, and fingers comprise a multitude of small muscles, tendons, and ligaments. Do not overstretch this area by applying too much force too quickly.

Complementary stretch
B11.

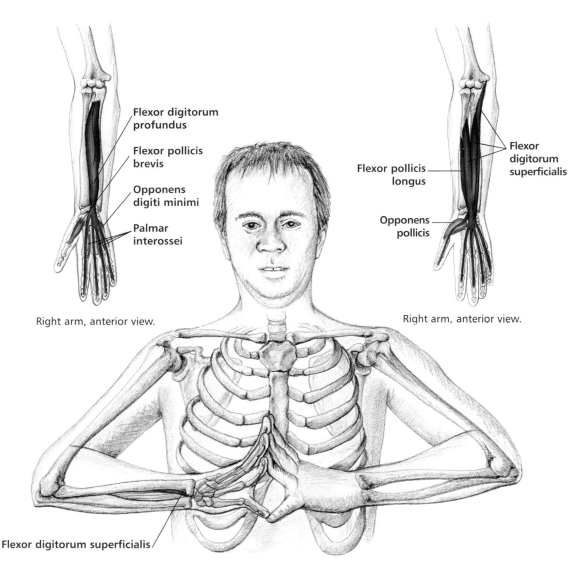

Right arm, anterior view.

Flexor digitorum profundus

Flexor pollicis brevis

Opponens digiti minimi

Palmar interossei

Flexor pollicis longus

Flexor digitorum superficialis

Opponens pollicis

Right arm, anterior view.

Flexor digitorum superficialis

Technique
Place the tips of your fingers together and push your palms towards each other.

Muscles being stretched
Primary muscles: Flexor digitorum superficialis. Flexor digitorum profundus. Flexor pollicis longus. Flexor pollicis brevis.
Secondary muscles: Opponens pollicis. Opponens digiti minimi. Palmar interossei.

Sports that benefit from this stretch
Basketball. Netball. Cricket. Baseball. Softball. Ice hockey. Field hockey. Martial arts. Tennis. Badminton. Squash. Rowing. Canoeing. Kayaking. Swimming. Athletics field events. Volleyball. Wrestling.

Sports injury where stretch may be useful
Tennis elbow. Golfer's elbow. Thrower's elbow. Wrist sprain. Wrist dislocation. Wrist tendonitis. Carpal tunnel syndrome. Ulnar tunnel syndrome.

Common problems and more information for performing this stretch correctly
The forearms, wrists, and fingers comprise a multitude of small muscles, tendons, and ligaments. Do not overstretch this area by applying too much force too quickly.

Complementary stretch
B13.

B15: THUMB STRETCH

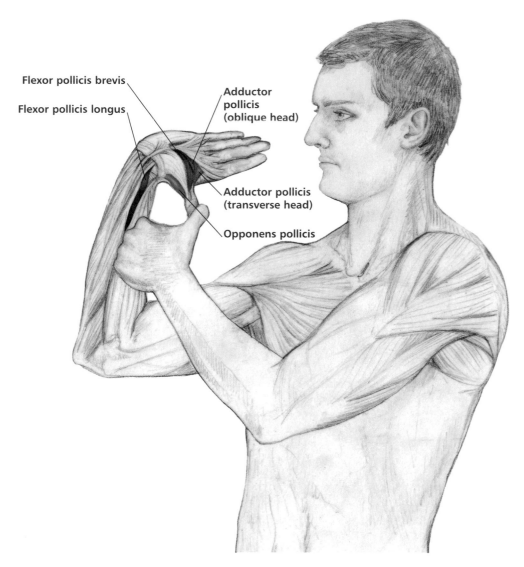

Flexor pollicis brevis

Flexor pollicis longus

Adductor pollicis (oblique head)

Adductor pollicis (transverse head)

Opponens pollicis

Technique
Start with your fingers pointing up and your thumb out to one side, then use your other hand to pull your thumb down.

Muscles being stretched
Primary muscles: Flexor pollicis longus. Flexor pollicis brevis.
Secondary muscles: Adductor pollicis. Opponens pollicis.

Sports that benefit from this stretch
Basketball. Netball. Cricket. Baseball. Softball. Ice hockey. Field hockey. Martial arts. Tennis. Badminton. Squash. Rowing. Canoeing. Kayaking. Swimming. Cricket. Baseball. Field events. Volleyball. Wrestling.

Sports injury where stretch may be useful
Tennis elbow. Golfer's elbow. Thrower's elbow. Wrist sprain. Wrist dislocation. Wrist tendonitis. Carpal tunnel syndrome. Ulnar tunnel syndrome.

Common problems and more information for performing this stretch correctly
The palm and thumb comprise a multitude of small muscles, tendons, and ligaments. Do not overstretch this area by applying too much force too quickly.

Complementary stretches
B12, B14.

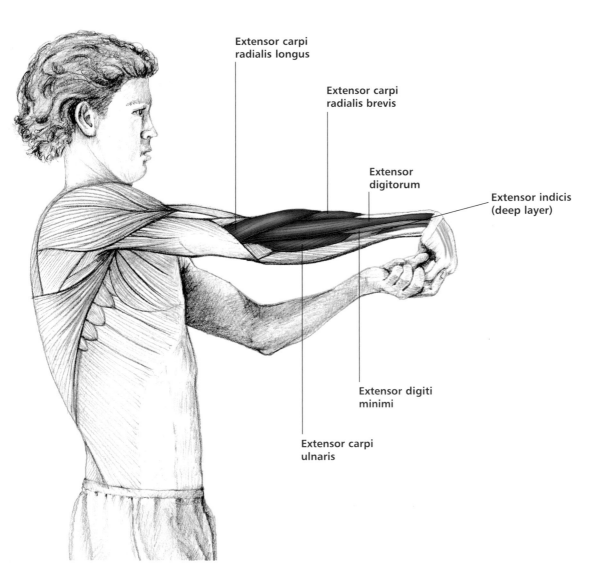

Extensor carpi
radialis longus

Extensor carpi
radialis brevis

Extensor
digitorum

Extensor indicis
(deep layer)

Extensor digiti
minimi

Extensor carpi
ulnaris

Technique
Hold on to your fingers while straightening
your arm. Pull your fingers towards your body.

Muscles being stretched
Primary muscles: Extensor carpi ulnaris.
Extensor carpi radialis longus and brevis.
Extensor digitorum.
Secondary muscles: Extensor digiti minimi.
Extensor indicis.

Sports that benefit from this stretch
Basketball. Netball. Cricket. Baseball. Softball.
Ice hockey. Field hockey. Martial arts. Tennis.
Badminton. Squash. Rowing. Canoeing.
Kayaking. Swimming. Athletics throwing field
events. Volleyball. Wrestling.

Sports injury where stretch may be useful
Tennis elbow. Golfer's elbow. Thrower's elbow.
Wrist sprain. Wrist dislocation. Wrist tendonitis.
Carpal tunnel syndrome. Ulnar tunnel
syndrome.

Common problems and more information for performing this stretch correctly
The forearms, wrists, and fingers comprise a
multitude of small muscles, tendons, and
ligaments. Do not overstretch this area by
applying too much force too quickly.

Complementary stretch
B17.

B17: ROTATING WRIST STRETCH

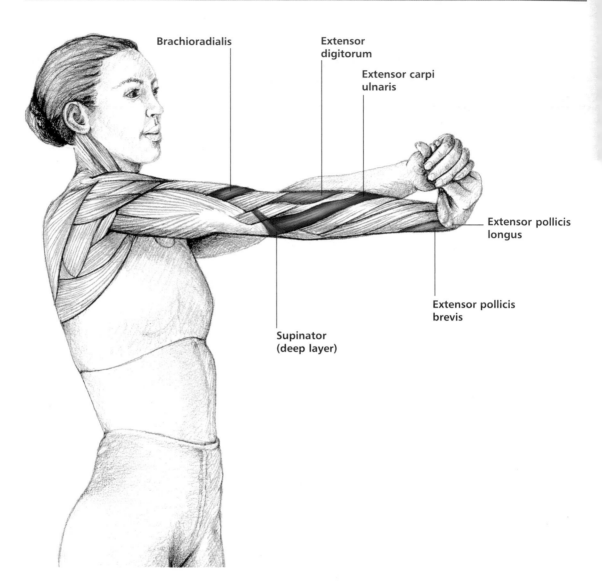

Brachioradialis

Extensor digitorum

Extensor carpi ulnaris

Extensor pollicis longus

Extensor pollicis brevis

Supinator (deep layer)

Technique
Place one arm straight out in front and parallel to the ground. Rotate your wrist down and outwards and then use your other hand to further rotate your hand upwards.

Muscles being stretched
Primary muscles: Brachioradialis. Extensor carpi ulnaris. Supinator.
Secondary muscles: Extensor digitorum. Extensor pollicis longus and brevis.

Sports that benefit from this stretch
Basketball. Netball. Cricket. Baseball. Softball. Ice hockey. Field hockey. Martial arts. Tennis. Badminton. Squash. Rowing. Canoeing. Kayaking. Swimming. Athletics throwing field events. Volleyball. Wrestling.

Sports injury where stretch may be useful
Tennis elbow. Golfer's elbow. Thrower's elbow. Wrist sprain. Wrist dislocation. Wrist tendonitis. Carpal tunnel syndrome. Ulnar tunnel syndrome.

Common problems and more information for performing this stretch correctly
The forearms, wrists, and fingers comprise a multitude of small muscles, tendons, and ligaments. Do not overstretch this area by applying too much force too quickly.

Complementary stretch
B16.

5 Stomach

The anterior abdominal wall muscles occur between the ribs and the pelvis, encircling the internal organs, and act to support the trunk, permit movement (primarily flex and rotate the lumbar spine), and support the lower back. There are three layers of muscle, with fibers running in the same direction as the corresponding three layers of muscle in the thoracic wall. The deepest layer consists of the **transversus abdominis**, whose fibers run approximately horizontally. Transversus abdominis spans around the trunk to attach into the *thoraco-lumbar fascia*, a thick connective tissue sheath, that helps to stabilise the trunk and pelvis when muscles connecting into it are under tension. The middle layer comprises the **internal oblique**, whose fibers are crossed by the outermost layer known as the **external oblique**, forming a pattern of fibers resembling a St. Andrew's cross. Overlying these three layers is the **rectus abdominis**, which runs vertically, on either side of the midline of the abdomen, and is associated with the *six-pack* muscles seen in conditioned athletes. Rectus abdominis is active in trunk flexion, bringing the rib cage closer to the pubic bone, for example in the crunch or sit-up. Like the other abdominals, it acts as a stabilising muscle, and also acts as a restraint to hyperextension in the lumbar vertebrae.

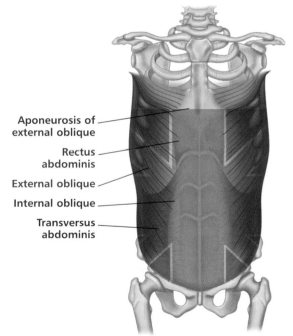

Aponeurosis of external oblique

Rectus abdominis

External oblique

Internal oblique

Transversus abdominis

Sports that benefit from these stomach stretches include: basketball and netball; batting sports like cricket, baseball and softball; boxing; contact sports like football, gridiron and rugby; golf; hiking, backpacking, mountaineering, and orienteering; ice hockey and field hockey; ice-skating, roller-skating, and inline skating; martial arts; rowing, canoeing, and kayaking; running, track, and cross-country; running sports like soccer, American football (gridiron), and rugby; snow skiing and water skiing; surfing; walking and race walking; wrestling.

C01: ON ELBOWS STOMACH STRETCH

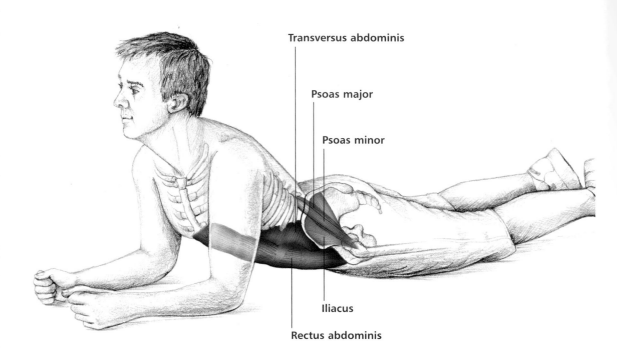

Transversus abdominis

Psoas major

Psoas minor

Iliacus

Rectus abdominis

Technique
Lie face down and bring your hands close to your shoulders. Keep your hips on the ground, look forward, and rise up onto your elbows.

Muscles being stretched
Primary muscles: Transversus abdominis. Rectus abdominis.
Secondary muscles: Psoas major and minor. Iliacus.

Sports that benefit from this stretch
Basketball. Netball. Cricket. Baseball. Softball. Boxing. Golf. Hiking. Backpacking. Mountaineering. Orienteering. Ice hockey. Field hockey. Ice-skating. Roller-skating. Inline skating. Martial arts. Rowing. Canoeing. Kayaking. Running. Track. Cross-country. American football (gridiron). Soccer. Rugby. Snow skiing. Water skiing. Surfing. Walking. Race walking. Wrestling.

Sports injury where stretch may be useful
Abdominal muscle strain.

Common problems and more information for performing this stretch correctly
For most people who spend their day in a seated position, (office workers, drivers, etc.) the muscles in the front of the body can become extremely tight and inflexible. Exercise caution when performing this stretch for the first time and allow plenty of rest time between each repetition.

Complementary stretch
C03.

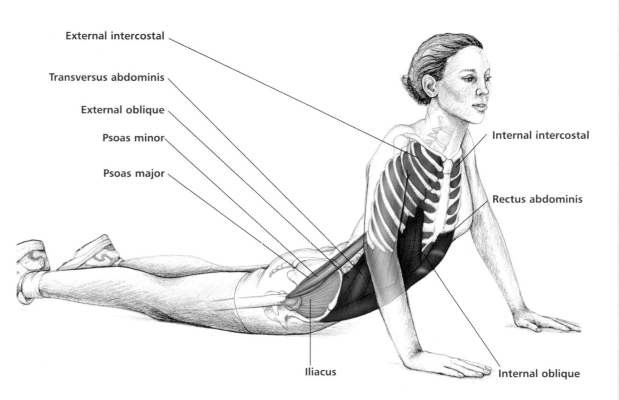

External intercostal

Transversus abdominis

External oblique

Psoas minor

Psoas major

Internal intercostal

Rectus abdominis

Iliacus

Internal oblique

Technique
Lie face down and bring your hands close to your shoulders. Keep your hips on the ground, look forward, and rise up by straightening your arms.

Muscles being stretched
Primary muscles: External and internal intercostals. External and internal obliques. Transversus abdominis. Rectus abdominis.
Secondary muscles: Psoas major and minor. Iliacus.

Sports that benefit from this stretch
Basketball. Netball. Cricket. Baseball. Softball. Boxing. Golf. Hiking. Backpacking. Mountaineering. Orienteering. Ice hockey. Field hockey. Ice-skating. Roller-skating. Inline skating. Martial arts. Rowing. Canoeing. Kayaking. Running. Track. Cross-country. American football (gridiron). Soccer. Rugby. Snow skiing. Water skiing. Surfing. Walking. Race walking. Wrestling.

Sports injury where stretch may be useful
Abdominal muscle strain. Hip flexor strain. Iliopsoas tendonitis.

Common problems and more information for performing this stretch correctly
For most people who spend their day in a seated position, (office workers, drivers, etc.) the muscles in the front of the body can become extremely tight and inflexible. Exercise caution when performing this stretch for the first time and allow plenty of rest time between each repetition.

Complementary stretch
C03.

C03: ROTATING STOMACH STRETCH

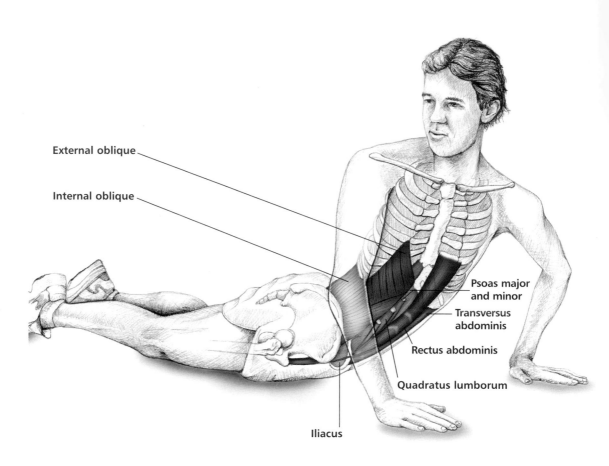

External oblique

Internal oblique

Psoas major and minor

Transversus abdominis

Rectus abdominis

Quadratus lumborum

Iliacus

Technique
Lie face down and bring your hands close to your shoulders. Keep your hips on the ground, look forward, and rise up by straightening your arms. Then slowly bend one arm and rotate that shoulder towards the ground.

Muscles being stretched
Primary muscles: External and internal obliques. Transversus abdominis. Rectus abdominis. Secondary muscles: Quadratus lumborum. Psoas major and minor. Iliacus.

Sports that benefit from this stretch
Basketball. Netball. Cricket. Baseball. Softball. Boxing. Golf. Hiking. Backpacking. Mountaineering. Orienteering. Ice hockey. Field hockey. Ice-skating. Roller-skating. Inline skating. Martial arts. Rowing. Canoeing. Kayaking. Running. Track. Cross-country. American football (gridiron). Soccer. Rugby. Snow skiing. Water skiing. Surfing. Walking. Race walking. Wrestling.

Sports injury where stretch may be useful
Abdominal muscle strain. Hip flexor strain. Iliopsoas tendonitis.

Common problems and more information for performing this stretch correctly
For most people who spend their day in a seated position, (office workers, drivers, etc.) the muscles in the front of the body can become extremely tight and inflexible. Exercise caution when performing this stretch for the first time and allow plenty of rest time between each repetition.

Complementary stretch
C06.

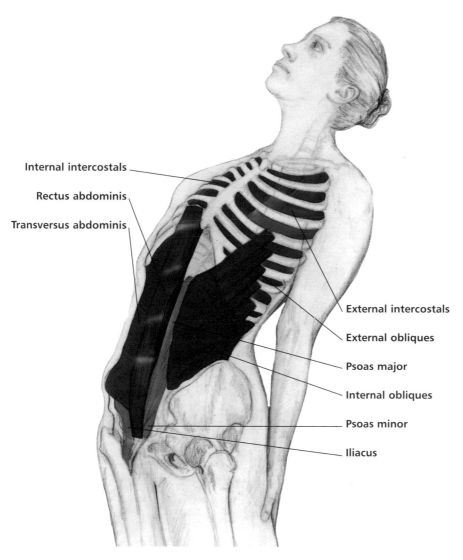

Internal intercostals

Rectus abdominis

Transversus abdominis

External intercostals

External obliques

Psoas major

Internal obliques

Psoas minor

Iliacus

Technique
Stand upright with your feet shoulder-width apart and place your hands on your buttocks for support. Look upwards and slowly lean backwards at the waist.

Muscles being stretched
Primary muscles: External and internal intercostals. External and internal obliques. Transversus abdominis. Rectus abdominis. Secondary muscles: Psoas major and minor. Iliacus.

Sports that benefit from this stretch
Basketball. Netball. Cricket. Baseball. Softball. Boxing. Golf. Hiking. Backpacking. Mountaineering. Orienteering. Ice hockey. Field hockey. Ice-skating. Roller-skating. Inline skating. Martial arts. Rowing. Canoeing. Kayaking. Running. Track. Cross-country. American football (gridiron). Soccer. Rugby. Snow skiing. Water skiing. Surfing. Walking. Race walking. Wrestling.

Sports injury where stretch may be useful
Abdominal muscle strain. Hip flexor strain. Iliopsoas tendonitis.

Common problems and more information for performing this stretch correctly
Do not perform this stretch if you suffer from lower back pain or have sustained an injury to your lower back. Exercise caution when performing for the first time and allow plenty of rest time between each repetition of this stretch.

Complementary stretch
C02.

C05: STANDING LEAN-BACK SIDE STOMACH STRETCH

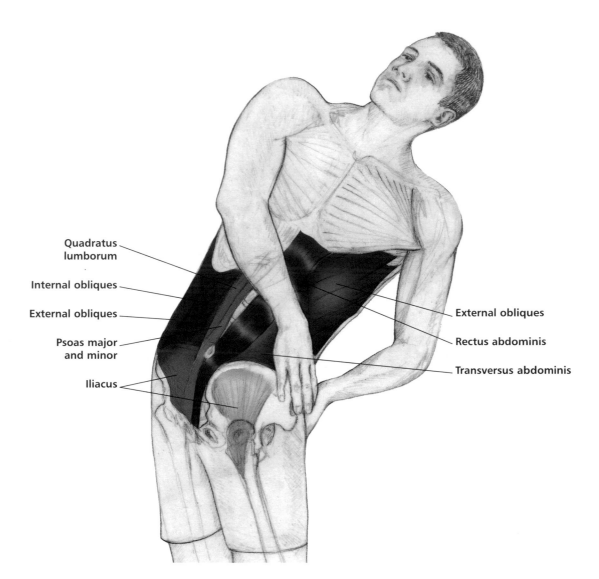

Quadratus lumborum

Internal obliques

External obliques

Psoas major and minor

Iliacus

External obliques

Rectus abdominis

Transversus abdominis

Technique
Stand upright with your feet shoulder-width apart and place one hand on your buttocks. Look up and slowly lean backwards at the waist, then reach over with your opposite hand and rotate at the waist.

Muscles being stretched
Primary muscles: External and internal obliques. Transversus abdominis. Rectus abdominis. Secondary muscles: Quadatus lumborum. Psoas major and minor. Iliacus.

Sports that benefit from this stretch
Basketball. Netball. Cricket. Baseball. Softball. Boxing. Golf. Hiking. Backpacking. Mountaineering. Orienteering. Ice hockey. Field hockey. Ice-skating. Roller-skating. Inline skating. Martial arts. Rowing. Canoeing. Kayaking. Running. Track. Cross-country. Football. Soccer. American football (gridiron). Rugby. Snow skiing. Water skiing. Surfing. Walking. Race walking. Wrestling.

Sports injury where stretch may be useful
Abdominal muscle strain. Hip flexor strain. Iliopsoas tendonitis.

Common problems and more information for performing this stretch correctly
Do not perform this stretch if you suffer from lower back pain or have sustained an injury to your lower back. Exercise caution when performing for the first time and allow plenty of rest time between each repetition of this stretch.

Complementary stretch
C03.

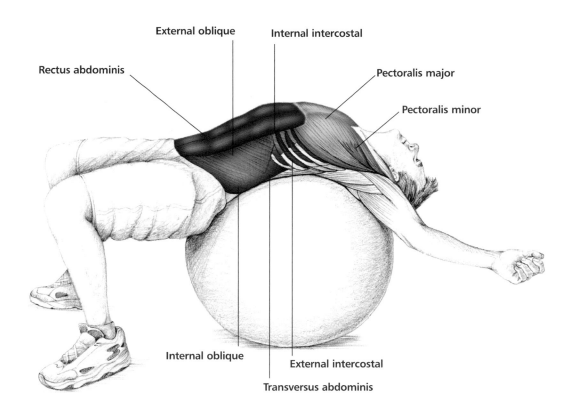

Rectus abdominis

External oblique

Internal intercostal

Pectoralis major

Pectoralis minor

Internal oblique

External intercostal

Transversus abdominis

Technique
Sit on a Swiss ball and slowly roll the ball forward while leaning back. Allow your back and shoulders to rest on the ball and your arms to hang to each side.

Muscles being stretched
Primary muscles: External and internal intercostals. External and internal obliques. Transversus abdominis. Rectus abdominis. Secondary muscles: Pectoralis major and minor.

Sports that benefit from this stretch
Basketball. Netball. Cricket. Baseball. Softball. Boxing. Golf. Hiking. Backpacking. Mountaineering. Orienteering. Ice hockey. Field hockey. Ice-skating. Roller-skating. Inline skating. Martial arts. Rowing. Canoeing. Kayaking. Running. Track. Cross-country. American football (gridiron). Soccer. Rugby. Snow skiing. Water skiing. Surfing. Walking. Race walking. Wrestling.

Sports injury where stretch may be useful
Abdominal muscle strain. Chest strain. Pectoral muscle insertion inflammation.

Common problems and more information for performing this stretch correctly
For most people who spend their day in a seated position, (office workers, drivers, etc.) the muscles in the front of the body can become extremely tight and inflexible. Exercise caution when performing this stretch for the first time and allow plenty of rest time between each repetition.

Complementary stretch
C02.

6

Back and Sides
(Upper, Middle, and Lower)

The muscles around the spine, and the broader area of the back, are primarily responsible for stabilising the spinal column and keeping the back in an upright position. The muscles of the back and sides allow the upper body and spine to move in flexion, lateral flexion, extension, hyperextension, and rotation.

Latissimus dorsi, the broadest muscle of the back, is one of the chief climbing muscles, since it pulls the shoulders downwards and backwards, and pulls the trunk up to the fixed arms. It is therefore heavily used in sports such as climbing, gymnastics (in particular rings and parallel bars), swimming, and rowing. The **rhomboid** muscles are situated between the scapula and vertebral column, and are so named because of their shape (rhombus); major being larger than minor. **Quadratus lumborum** runs across the waist from the iliac crest to the pelvis and iliolumbar ligament to the lowest rib and transverse processes of L1 to L4. Its action is to side bend the trunk, and also to resist the trunk being pulled sideways in the opposite direction.

The lower **external intercostal** muscles may blend with the fibers of external oblique, which overlap them, thus effectively forming one continuous sheet of muscle, with the external intercostal fibers seemingly stranded between the ribs. **Internal intercostal** fibers lie deep to, and run obliquely across, the external intercostals. There are eleven external and internal intercostals on each side of the rib cage.

Erector spinae, also called sacrospinalis, comprises three sets of muscles organised in parallel columns. From lateral to medial, they are: iliocostalis, longissimus, and spinalis. Longissimus is the intermediate part of the erector spinae. It may be subdivided into thoracis, cervicis, and capitis portions. The spinalis is the most medial part of the erector spinae. It may also be subdivided into thoracis, cervicis, and capitis portions. The **transversospinalis** muscles are a composite of three small muscle groups situated deep to erector spinae. However, unlike erector spinae, each group lies successively deeper from the surface rather than side-by-side. The muscle groups are, from more superficial to deep: semispinalis, multifidus, and rotatores. Their fibers generally extend upward and medially from transverse processes to higher spinous processes. **Multifidus** is the part of the transversospinalis group that lies in the furrow between the vertebrae of the spine and their transverse processes. It lies deep to semispinalis and erector spinae. **Rotatores** are the deepest layer of the transversospinalis group.

Interspinales are short and insignificant muscles positioned on either side of the interspinous ligament. Like the interspinales, the **intertransversarii** are also short and insignificant muscles. The cervical and thoracic regions encompass intertransversarii anteriores and intertransversarii posteriores, and the lumbar region encompasses intertransversarii laterales and intertransversarii mediales.

Sports that benefit from these back and side stretches include: archery; basketball and netball; batting sports like cricket, baseball, and softball; boxing; contact sports like football, rugby, and gridiron; cycling; golf; hiking, backpacking, mountaineering, and orienteering; ice hockey and field hockey; ice-skating, roller-skating, and inline skating; martial arts; racquet sports like tennis, badminton, and squash; rowing, canoeing, and kayaking; running, track, and cross-country; running sports like soccer, American football (gridiron), and rugby; snow skiing and water skiing; surfing; swimming; throwing sports like cricket, baseball, and field events; volleyball; walking and race walking; wrestling.

D01: REACHING FORWARD UPPER BACK STRETCH

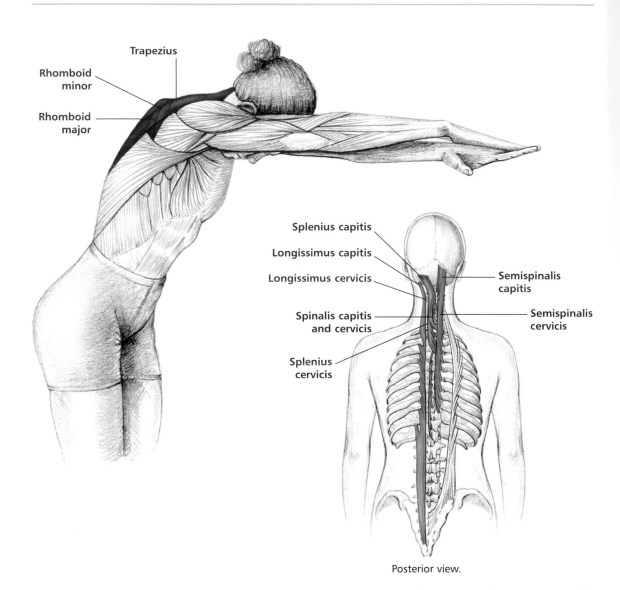

Posterior view.

Technique
Stand with your arms out in front and crossed over. Push your hands forward as far as possible and let your head fall forward.

Muscles being stretched
Primary muscles: Trapezius. Rhomboids. Secondary muscles: Semispinalis capitis and cervicis. Spinalis capitis and cervicis. Longissimus capitis and cervicis. Splenius capitis and cervicis.

Sports that benefit from this stretch
Archery. Boxing. Cycling. Golf. Tennis. Badminton. Squash. Rowing. Canoeing. Kayaking. Snow skiing. Water skiing. Swimming.

Sports injury where stretch may be useful
Neck muscle strain. Whiplash (neck sprain). Cervical nerve stretch syndrome. Wryneck (acute torticollis). Upper back muscle strain. Upper back ligament sprain.

Additional information for performing this stretch correctly
Concentrate on reaching forward with your hands and separating your shoulder-blades.

Complementary stretch
D05.

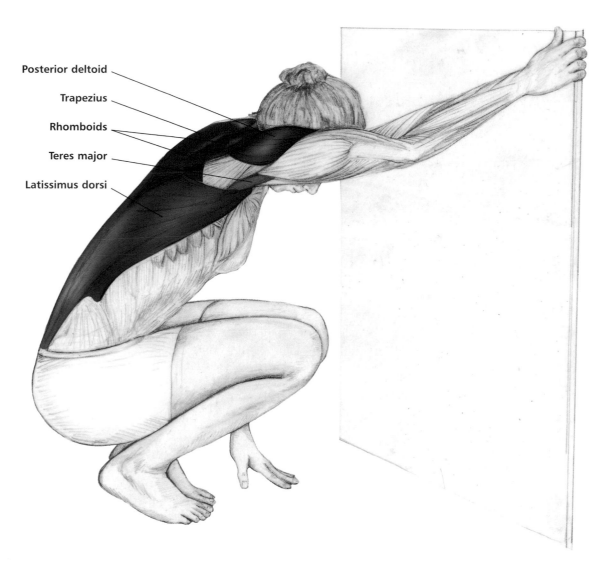

Posterior deltoid

Trapezius

Rhomboids

Teres major

Latissimus dorsi

Technique
Sit in a squatting position while facing a door edge or pole, then hold onto the door edge with one hand and lean backwards away from the door.

Muscles being stretched
Primary muscles: Trapezius. Rhomboids. Latissimus dorsi. Posterior deltoid. Secondary muscle: Teres major.

Sports that benefit from this stretch
Archery. Boxing. Cycling. Golf. Tennis. Badminton. Squash. Rowing. Canoeing. Kayaking. Snow skiing. Water skiing. Swimming.

Sports injury where stretch may be useful
Neck muscle strain. Whiplash (neck sprain). Cervical nerve stretch syndrome. Wryneck (acute torticollis). Upper back muscle strain. Upper back ligament sprain. Impingement syndrome. Rotator cuff tendonitis. Shoulder bursitis. Frozen shoulder (adhesive capsulitis).

Common problems and more information for performing this stretch correctly
Lean backwards and let the weight of your body do the stretching. Relax your upper back, allowing it to round out and your shoulder-blades to separate.

Complementary stretches
D01, A08.

D03: REACH-UP BACK STRETCH

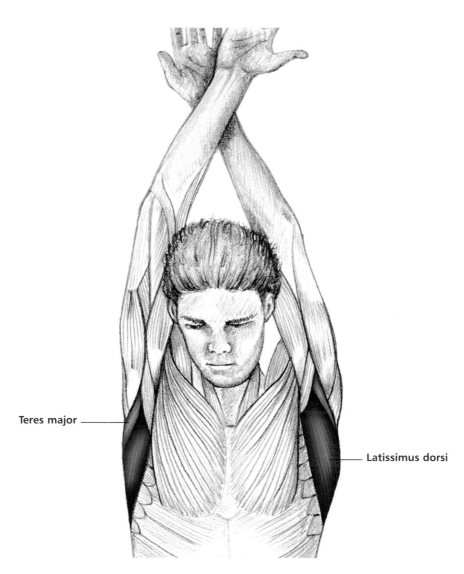

Teres major

Latissimus dorsi

Technique
Stand with your arms crossed over and then raise them above your head. Reach up as far as you can.

Muscles being stretched
Primary muscle: Latissimus dorsi.
Secondary muscle: Teres major.

Sports that benefit from this stretch
Basketball. Netball. Swimming. Volleyball.

Sports injury where stretch may be useful
Neck muscle strain. Whiplash (neck sprain). Cervical nerve stretch syndrome. Wryneck (acute torticollis). Upper back muscle strain. Upper back ligament sprain.

Additional information for performing this stretch correctly
Let your head fall forward so that your arms can reach straight upwards without touching your head.

Complementary stretch
D04.

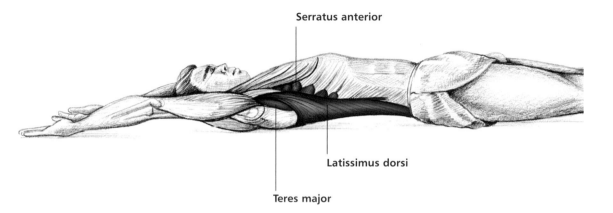

Serratus anterior

Latissimus dorsi

Teres major

Technique
Lie on your back and extend your arms behind you. Raise your toes and then lengthen your body as much as you can.

Muscles being stretched
Primary muscles: Serratus anterior. Latissimus dorsi.
Secondary muscle: Teres major.

Sports that benefit from this stretch
Basketball. Netball. Swimming. Volleyball.

Sports injury where stretch may be useful
Back muscle strain. Back ligament sprain.

Additional information for performing this stretch correctly
Concentrate on extending your legs by pushing with your heels, rather than your toes.

Complementary stretch
D03.

D05: SITTING BENT-OVER BACK STRETCH

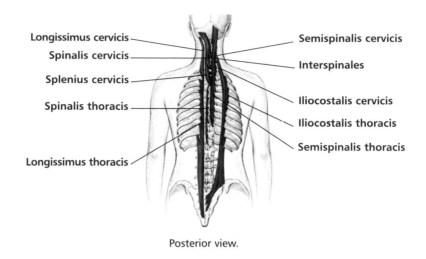

Longissimus cervicis
Spinalis cervicis
Splenius cervicis
Spinalis thoracis
Longissimus thoracis

Semispinalis cervicis
Interspinales
Iliocostalis cervicis
Iliocostalis thoracis
Semispinalis thoracis

Posterior view.

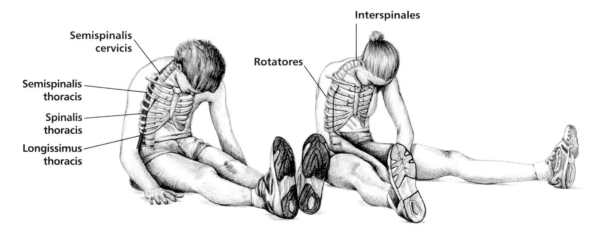

Semispinalis cervicis
Semispinalis thoracis
Spinalis thoracis
Longissimus thoracis

Interspinales
Rotatores

Technique

Sit on the ground with your legs straight out in front or at 45 degrees apart. Keep your toes pointing upwards and rest your arms by your side or on your lap. Relax your back and neck and then let your head and chest fall forward.

Muscles being stretched

Primary muscles: Semispinalis cervicis and thoracis. Spinalis cervicis and thoracis. Longissimus cervicis and thoracis. Splenius cervicis. Iliocostalis cervicis and thoracis. Secondary muscles: Interspinales. Rotatores.

Sports that benefit from this stretch

Cricket. Baseball. Softball. American football (gridiron). Rugby. Cycling. Golf. Hiking. Backpacking. Mountaineering. Orienteering. Ice hockey. Field hockey. Tennis. Badminton. Squash. Rowing. Canoeing. Kayaking. Swimming.

Sports injury where stretch may be useful

Neck muscle strain. Whiplash (neck sprain). Cervical nerve stretch syndrome. Wryneck (acute torticollis). Back muscle strain. Back ligament sprain.

Common problems and more information for performing this stretch correctly

Where this stretch is primarily felt will depend on where you are most tight. Some people will feel most tension in the neck and upper back, whereas others will feel most tension in the lower back and hamstrings. This stretch gives a good indication of where you need to improve your flexibility.

Complementary stretch

D01.

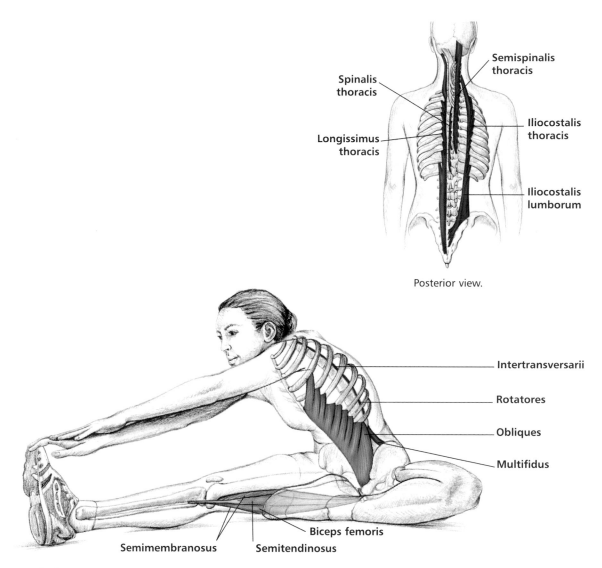

Posterior view.

Technique
Sit with one leg straight out to the side and your toes pointing up. Then bring your other foot up to your knee and let your head fall forward. Reach towards the outside of your toes with both hands.

Muscles being stretched
Primary muscles: Semispinalis thoracis. Spinalis thoracis. Longissimus thoracis. Iliocostalis thoracis. Iliocostalis lumborum. Intertransversarii. Rotatores. Multifidus.
Secondary muscles: Obliques. Semimembranosus. Semitendinosus. Biceps femoris.

Sports that benefit from this stretch
Cricket. Baseball. Softball. Boxing. American football (gridiron). Rugby. Cycling. Golf. Hiking. Backpacking. Mountaineering. Orienteering. Ice hockey. Field hockey. Tennis. Badminton. Squash. Rowing. Canoeing. Kayaking. Swimming. Running. Walking. Race walking.

Sports injury where stretch may be useful
Neck muscle strain. Whiplash (neck sprain). Cervical nerve stretch syndrome. Wryneck (acute torticollis). Back muscle strain. Back ligament sprain.

Additional information for performing this stretch correctly
It is not important to be able to touch your toes. Simply reaching towards the outside of your toes is sufficient.

Complementary stretch
D21.

D07: STANDING KNEE-TO-CHEST STRETCH

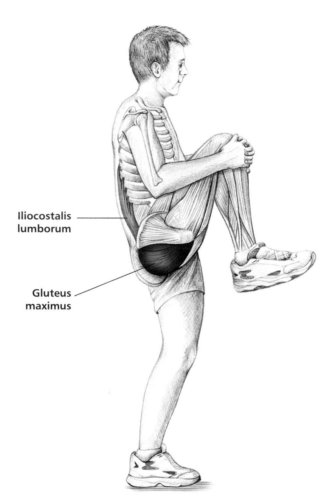

Iliocostalis lumborum

Gluteus maximus

Technique
While standing, use your hands to bring one knee into your chest.

Muscles being stretched
Primary muscle: Gluteus maximus.
Secondary muscle: Iliocostalis lumborum.

Sports that benefit from this stretch
Basketball. Netball. Cycling. Hiking. Backpacking. Mountaineering. Orienteering. Ice hockey. Field hockey. Ice-skating. Roller-skating. Inline skating. Martial arts. Running. Track. Cross-country. American football (gridiron). Soccer. Rugby. Snow skiing. Water skiing. Surfing. Walking. Race walking.

Sports injury where stretch may be useful
Lower back muscle strain. Lower back ligament sprain. Hamstring strain.

Additional information for performing this stretch correctly
Make sure you have good balance when performing this stretch, or lean against an object to stop yourself from falling over.

Complementary stretch
D08.

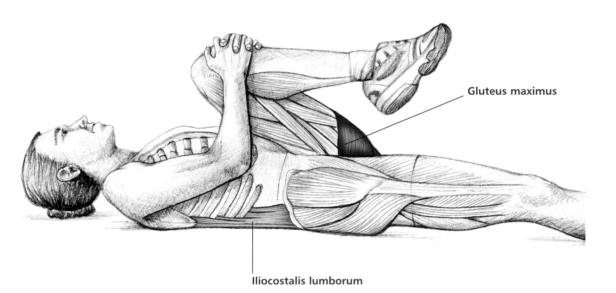

Gluteus maximus

Iliocostalis lumborum

Technique
Lie on your back and keep one leg flat on the ground. Use your hands to bring your other knee into your chest.

Muscles being stretched
Primary muscle: Gluteus maximus.
Secondary muscle: Iliocostalis lumborum.

Sports that benefit from this stretch
Basketball. Netball. Cycling. Hiking. Backpacking. Mountaineering. Orienteering. Ice hockey. Field hockey. Ice-skating. Roller-skating. Inline skating. Martial arts. Running. Track. Cross-country. American football (gridiron). Soccer. Rugby. Snow skiing. Water skiing. Surfing. Walking. Race walking.

Sports injury where stretch may be useful
Lower back muscle strain. Lower back ligament sprain. Hamstring strain.

Additional information for performing this stretch correctly
Rest your back, head, and neck on the ground and do not be tempted to raise your head off the ground.

Complementary stretch
D08.

D09: LYING DOUBLE KNEE-TO-CHEST STRETCH

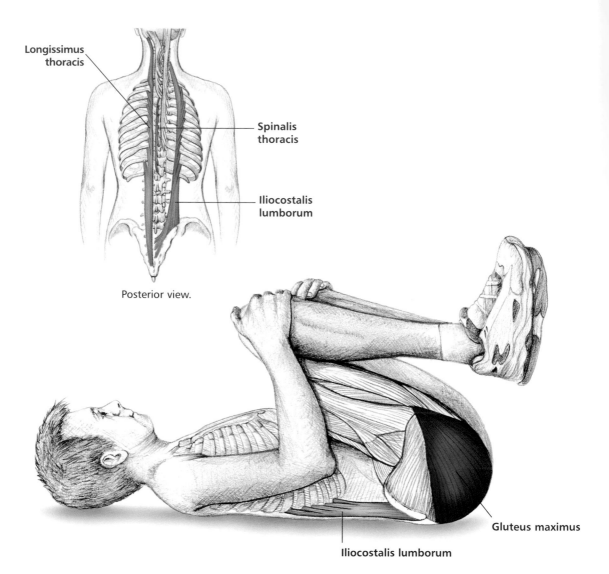

Posterior view.

Longissimus thoracis

Spinalis thoracis

Iliocostalis lumborum

Gluteus maximus

Iliocostalis lumborum

Technique
Lie on your back and use your hands to bring both knees into your chest.

Muscles being stretched
Primary muscle: Gluteus maximus.
Secondary muscles: Iliocostalis lumborum. Spinalis thoracis. Longissimus thoracis.

Sports that benefit from this stretch
Basketball. Netball. Cycling. Hiking. Backpacking. Mountaineering. Orienteering. Ice hockey. Field hockey. Ice-skating. Roller-skating. Inline skating. Martial arts. Running. Track. Cross-country. American football (gridiron). Soccer. Rugby. Snow skiing. Water skiing. Surfing. Walking. Race walking.

Sports injury where stretch may be useful
Lower back muscle strain. Lower back ligament sprain. Hamstring strain.

Additional information for performing this stretch correctly
Rest your back, head, and neck on the ground and don't be tempted to raise your head off the ground.

Complementary stretch
D07.

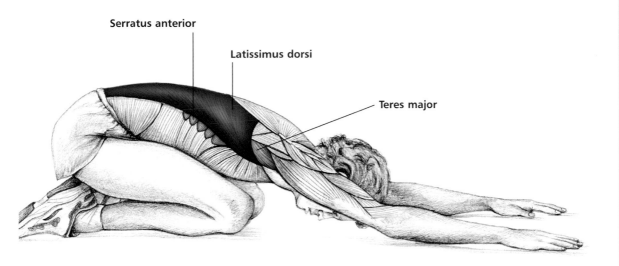

Serratus anterior

Latissimus dorsi

Teres major

Technique
Kneel on the ground and reach forward with your hands. Let your head fall forward and push your buttocks towards your feet.

Muscles being stretched
Primary muscle: Latissimus dorsi.
Secondary muscles: Teres major. Serratus anterior.

Sports that benefit from this stretch
Basketball. Netball. Swimming. Volleyball.

Sports injury where stretch may be useful
Lower back muscle strain. Lower back ligament sprain.

Additional information for performing this stretch correctly
Use your hands and fingers to walk your arms forward and extend this stretch, but do not lift your backside off your feet.

Complementary stretch
D04.

D11: KNEELING BACK-ARCH STRETCH

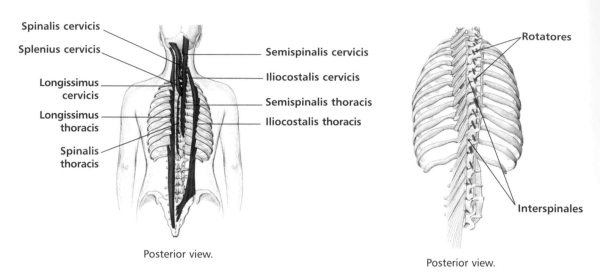

Spinalis cervicis
Splenius cervicis
Longissimus cervicis
Longissimus thoracis
Spinalis thoracis
Semispinalis cervicis
Iliocostalis cervicis
Semispinalis thoracis
Iliocostalis thoracis

Posterior view.

Rotatores
Interspinales

Posterior view.

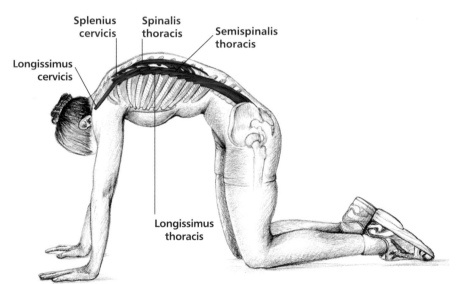

Splenius cervicis
Spinalis thoracis
Semispinalis thoracis
Longissimus cervicis
Longissimus thoracis

Technique
Kneel on your hands and knees. Let your head fall forwards and arch your back upwards.

Muscles being stretched
Primary muscles: Semispinalis cervicis and thoracis. Spinalis cervicis and thoracis. Longissimus cervicis and thoracis. Splenius cervicis. Iliocostalis cervicis and thoracis. Secondary muscles: Interspinales. Rotatores.

Sports that benefit from this stretch
Cricket. Baseball. Softball. Cycling. Golf. Hiking. Backpacking. Mountaineering. Orienteering. Ice hockey. Field hockey. Tennis. Badminton. Squash. Rowing. Canoeing. Kayaking. Running. Track. Cross-country. Soccer. American football (gridiron). Rugby. Swimming. Walking. Race walking.

Sports injury where stretch may be useful
Neck muscle strain. Whiplash (neck sprain). Cervical nerve stretch syndrome. Wryneck (acute torticollis). Back muscle strain. Back ligament sprain.

Common problems and more information for performing this stretch correctly
Perform this stretch slowly and deliberately, resting your weight evenly on both your knees and hands.

Complementary stretches
D05, D09.

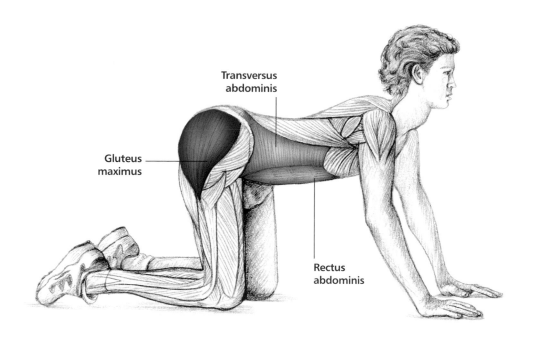

Transversus abdominis

Gluteus maximus

Rectus abdominis

Technique
Kneel on your hands and knees. Look up and let your back slump downwards.

Muscles being stretched
Primary muscle: Gluteus maximus.
Secondary muscles: Transversus abdominis. Rectus abdominis.

Sports that benefit from this stretch
Cricket. Baseball. Softball. Cycling. Golf. Hiking. Backpacking. Mountaineering. Orienteering. Ice hockey. Field hockey. Tennis. Badminton. Squash. Rowing. Canoeing. Kayaking. Running. Track. Cross-country. Soccer. American football (gridiron). Rugby. Swimming. Walking. Race walking.

Sports injury where stretch may be useful
Neck muscle strain. Whiplash (neck sprain). Cervical nerve stretch syndrome. Wryneck (acute torticollis). Back muscle strain. Back ligament sprain.

Common problems and more information for performing this stretch correctly
Perform this stretch slowly and deliberately, resting your weight evenly on both your knees and hands.

Complementary stretches
C02, C03.

D13: KNEELING BACK ROTATION STRETCH

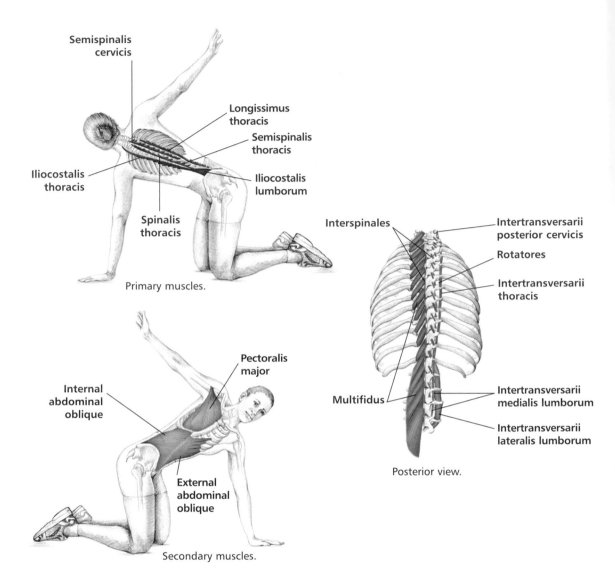

Primary muscles.

Secondary muscles.

Posterior view.

Technique
Kneel on the ground and raise one arm. Then rotate your shoulders and middle back while looking upwards.

Muscles being stretched
Primary muscles: Semispinalis thoracis. Spinalis thoracis. Longissimus thoracis. Iliocostalis thoracis. Iliocostalis lumborum. Multifidus. Rotatores. Intertransversarii. Interspinales. Secondary muscles: External and internal obliques. Pectoralis major.

Sports that benefit from this stretch
Archery. Basketball. Netball. Cricket. Baseball. Softball. Boxing. Cycling. Golf. Hiking. Backpacking. Mountaineering. Orienteering. Ice hockey. Field hockey. Ice-skating. Roller-skating. Inline skating. Martial arts. Tennis. Badminton. Squash. Rowing. Canoeing. Kayaking. Running. Track. Cross-country. American football (gridiron). Soccer. Rugby. Snow skiing. Water skiing. Surfing. Swimming. Athletics field events. Walking. Race walking. Wrestling.

Sports injury where stretch may be useful
Back muscle strain. Back ligament sprain. Abdominal muscle strain (obliques).

Additional information for performing this stretch correctly
Keep your arm pointing straight upward and follow your hand with your eyes. This will help to further extend the stretch into your neck.

Complementary stretch
D14.

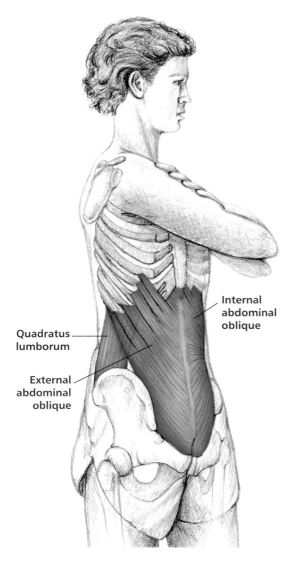

Quadratus lumborum

External abdominal oblique

Internal abdominal oblique

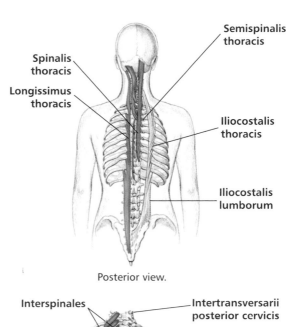

Spinalis thoracis

Longissimus thoracis

Semispinalis thoracis

Iliocostalis thoracis

Iliocostalis lumborum

Posterior view.

Interspinales

Multifidus

Intertransversarii posterior cervicis

Rotatores

Intertransversarii thoracis

Intertransversarii medialis lumborum

Intertransversarii lateralis lumborum

Posterior view.

Technique
Stand with your feet shoulder-width apart. Place your hands across your chest while keeping your back and shoulders upright. Slowly rotate your shoulders to one side.

Muscles being stretched
Primary muscles: Semispinalis thoracis. Spinalis thoracis. Longissimus thoracis. Iliocostalis thoracis. Iliocostalis lumborum. Multifidus. Rotatores. Intertransversarii. Interspinales. Secondary muscles: Quadratus lumborum. External and internal obliques.

Sports that benefit from this stretch
Archery. Basketball. Netball. Cricket. Baseball. Softball. Boxing. American football (gridiron). Rugby. Cycling. Golf. Hiking. Backpacking. Mountaineering. Orienteering. Ice hockey. Field hockey. Ice-skating. Roller-skating. Inline skating. Martial arts. Tennis. Badminton. Squash. Rowing. Canoeing. Kayaking. Water skiing. Surfing. Swimming. Running. Track. Cross-country. Soccer. Snow skiing. Athletic field events. Walking. Race walking. Wrestling.

Sports injury where stretch may be useful
Back muscle strain. Back ligament sprain. Abdominal muscle strain (obliques).

Additional information for performing this stretch correctly
To further extend this stretch use your hands to pull your upper body further around.

Complementary stretch
D16.

STRETCHES FOR THE BACK AND SIDES

D15: STANDING REACH-UP BACK ROTATION STRETCH

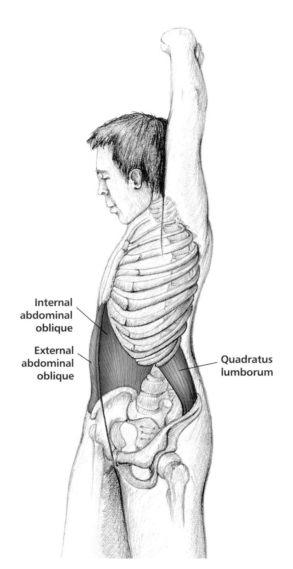

Internal abdominal oblique

External abdominal oblique

Quadratus lumborum

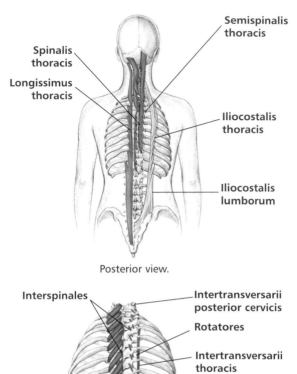

Spinalis thoracis

Longissimus thoracis

Semispinalis thoracis

Iliocostalis thoracis

Iliocostalis lumborum

Posterior view.

Interspinales

Intertransversarii posterior cervicis

Rotatores

Intertransversarii thoracis

Multifidus

Intertransversarii medialis lumborum

Intertransversarii lateralis lumborum

Posterior view.

Technique
Stand with your feet shoulder-width apart. Place your hands above your head while keeping your back and shoulders upright. Slowly rotate your shoulders to one side.

Muscles being stretched
Primary muscles: Semispinalis thoracis. Spinalis thoracis. Longissimus thoracis. Iliocostalis thoracis. Iliocostalis lumborum. Multifidus. Rotatores. Intertransversarii. Interspinales. Secondary muscles: Quadratus lumborum. External and internal obliques.

Sports that benefit from this stretch
Archery. Basketball. Netball. Cricket. Baseball. Softball. Boxing. American football (gridiron). Rugby. Cycling. Golf. Hiking. Backpacking. Mountaineering. Orienteering. Ice hockey. Field hockey. Ice-skating. Roller-skating. Inline skating. Martial arts. Tennis. Badminton. Squash. Rowing. Canoeing. Kayaking. Running. Track. Cross-country. Snow skiing. Water skiing. Surfing. Swimming. Athletics field events. Walking. Race walking. Wrestling.

Sports injury where stretch may be useful
Back muscle strain. Back ligament sprain. Abdominal muscle strain (obliques).

Common problems and more information for performing this stretch correctly
Lean back slightly to emphasize the *oblique* muscles. Do not perform if you suffer from lower back pain.

Complementary stretch
D13.

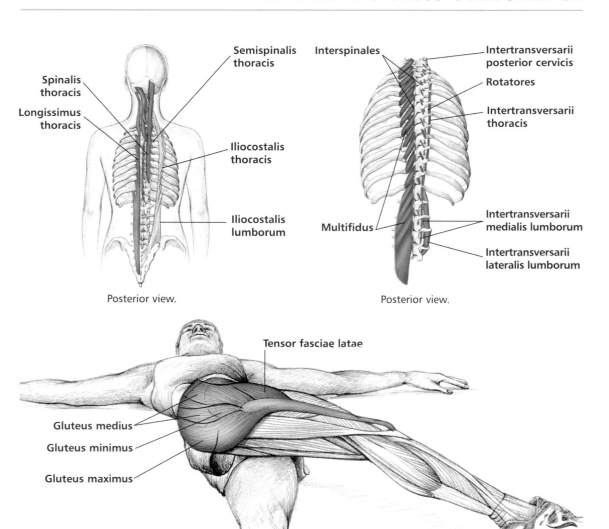

Semispinalis thoracis

Spinalis thoracis

Longissimus thoracis

Iliocostalis thoracis

Iliocostalis lumborum

Posterior view.

Interspinales

Intertransversarii posterior cervicis

Rotatores

Intertransversarii thoracis

Multifidus

Intertransversarii medialis lumborum

Intertransversarii lateralis lumborum

Posterior view.

Tensor fasciae latae

Gluteus medius

Gluteus minimus

Gluteus maximus

Technique
Lie on your back and cross one leg over the other. Keep your arms out to the side and both legs straight. Let your back and hips rotate with your leg.

Muscles being stretched
Primary muscles: Semispinalis thoracis. Spinalis thoracis. Longissimus thoracis. Iliocostalis thoracis. Iliocostalis lumborum. Multifidus. Rotatores. Intertransversarii. Interspinales. Secondary muscles: Gluteus maximus, medius, and minimus. Tensor fasciae latae.

Sports that benefit from this stretch
Cycling. Hiking. Backpacking. Mountaineering. Orienteering. Ice hockey. Field hockey. Ice-skating. Roller-skating. Inline skating. Martial arts. Running. Track. Cross-country. American football (gridiron). Soccer. Rugby. Snow skiing. Water skiing. Surfing. Walking. Race walking. Wrestling.

Sports injury where stretch may be useful
Lower back muscle strain. Lower back ligament sprain. Iliotibial band syndrome.

Additional information for performing this stretch correctly
Keep your shoulders on the ground and avoid lifting them during this stretch. Do not throw your leg over to the side; simply let the weight of your leg do most of the stretching for you.

Complementary stretch
D17.

D17: LYING KNEE ROLL-OVER STRETCH

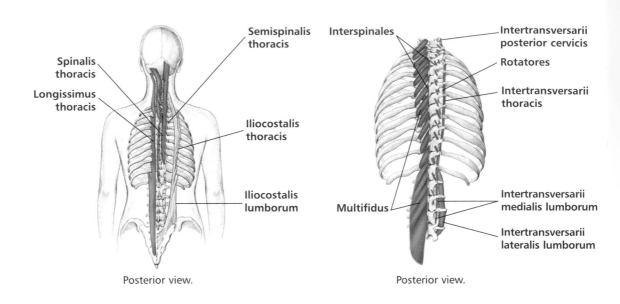

Posterior view.

Posterior view.

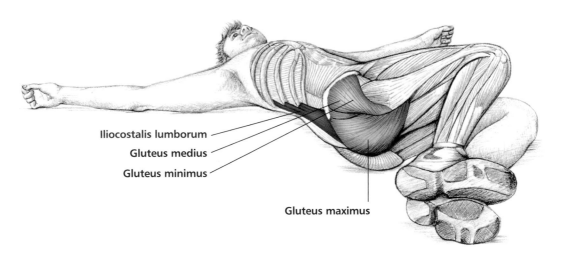

Technique
Lie on your back, keep your knees together and raise them slightly. Keep your arms out to the side and then let your back and hips rotate with your knees.

Muscles being stretched
Primary muscles: Semispinalis thoracis. Spinalis thoracis. Longissimus thoracis. Iliocostalis thoracis. Iliocostalis lumborum. Multifidus. Rotatores. Intertransversarii. Interspinales. Secondary muscles: Gluteus maximus, medius, and minimus.

Sports that benefit from this stretch
Cycling. Hiking. Backpacking. Mountaineering. Orienteering. Ice hockey. Field hockey. Ice-skating. Roller-skating. Inline skating. Martial arts. Running. Track. Cross-country. American football (gridiron). Soccer. Rugby. Snow skiing. Water skiing. Surfing. Walking. Race walking. Wrestling.

Sports injury where stretch may be useful
Lower back muscle strain. Lower back ligament sprain. Iliotibial band syndrome.

Additional information for performing this stretch correctly
Keep your shoulders on the ground and avoid lifting them during this stretch. Do not throw your legs over to the side; simply let the weight of your legs do most of the stretching for you.

Complementary stretch
D14.

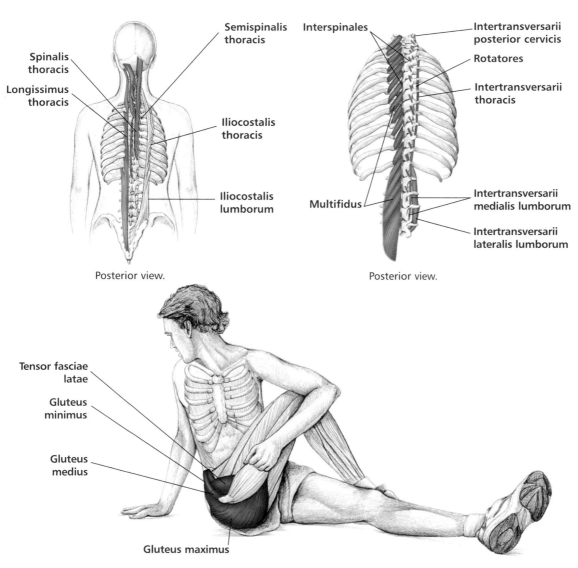

Semispinalis thoracis

Spinalis thoracis

Longissimus thoracis

Iliocostalis thoracis

Iliocostalis lumborum

Posterior view.

Interspinales

Intertransversarii posterior cervicis

Rotatores

Intertransversarii thoracis

Multifidus

Intertransversarii medialis lumborum

Intertransversarii lateralis lumborum

Posterior view.

Tensor fasciae latae

Gluteus minimus

Gluteus medius

Gluteus maximus

Technique
Sit with one leg straight and the other leg crossed over your knee. Turn your shoulders and put your arm onto your raised knee to help rotate your shoulders and back.

Muscles being stretched
Primary muscles: Gluteus maximus, medius, and minimus. Tensor fasciae latae.
Secondary muscles: Semispinalis thoracis. Spinalis thoracis. Longissimus thoracis. Iliocostalis thoracis. Iliocostalis lumborum. Multifidus. Rotatores. Intertransversarii. Interspinales.

Sports that benefit from this stretch
Cycling. Hiking. Backpacking. Mountaineering. Orienteering. Ice hockey. Field hockey. Ice-skating. Roller-skating. Inline skating. Martial arts. Running. Track. Cross-country. American football (gridiron). Soccer. Rugby. Snow skiing. Water skiing. Walking. Race walking. Wrestling.

Sports injury where stretch may be useful
Lower back muscle strain. Lower back ligament sprain. Abdominal muscle strain (obliques). Iliotibial band syndrome.

Additional information for performing this stretch correctly
Keep your hips straight and concentrate on rotating your lower back.

Complementary stretch
D16.

D19: SITTING KNEE-UP EXTENDED ROTATION STRETCH

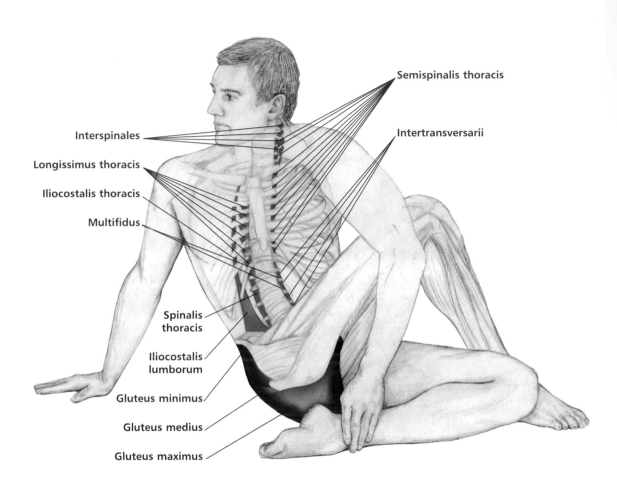

Interspinales

Longissimus thoracis

Iliocostalis thoracis

Multifidus

Spinalis thoracis

Iliocostalis lumborum

Gluteus minimus

Gluteus medius

Gluteus maximus

Semispinalis thoracis

Intertransversarii

Technique
Sit with one leg crossed under the other and the other foot crossed over your knee; then turn your shoulders and put your arm onto your raised knee to help rotate your shoulders and back.

Muscles being stretched
Primary muscles: Gluteus maximus, medius, and minimus.
Secondary muscles: Semispinalis thoracis. Spinalis thoracis. Longissimus thoracis. Iliocostalis thoracis. Iliocostalis lumborum. Multifidus. Rotatores. Intertransversarii. Interspinales.

Sports that benefit from this stretch
Cycling. Hiking. Backpacking. Mountaineering. Orienteering. Ice hockey. Field hockey. Ice-skating. Roller-skating. Inline skating. Martial arts. Running. Track. Cross-country. Soccer.

American football (gridiron). Rugby. Snow skiing. Water skiing. Walking. Race walking. Wrestling.

Sports injury where stretch may be useful
Lower back muscle strain. Lower back ligament sprain. Abdominal muscle strain (obliques). Iliotibial band syndrome.

Common problems and more information for performing this stretch correctly
Keep your hips straight and concentrate on rotating your lower back. This stretch also requires a good level of hip flexibility; do not perform if you experience pain or excessive tension in the hips.

Complementary stretches
D17, D21.

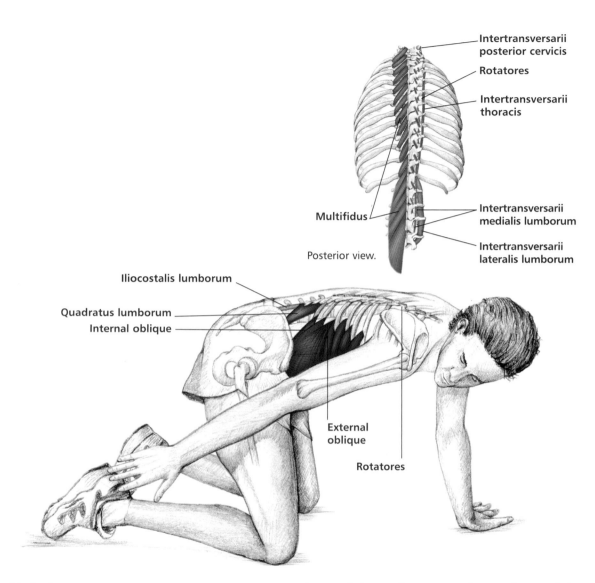

Intertransversarii posterior cervicis

Rotatores

Intertransversarii thoracis

Multifidus

Intertransversarii medialis lumborum

Intertransversarii lateralis lumborum

Posterior view.

Iliocostalis lumborum

Quadratus lumborum

Internal oblique

External oblique

Rotatores

Technique
Kneel on your hands and knees and then take one hand and reach around towards your ankle. Keep your back parallel to the ground.

Muscles being stretched
Primary muscles: Quadratus lumborum. External and internal obliques. Secondary muscles: Iliocostalis lumborum. Intertransversarii. Rotatores. Multifidus.

Sports that benefit from this stretch
Cricket. Baseball. Softball. Boxing. American football (gridiron). Rugby. Hiking. Backpacking. Mountaineering. Orienteering. Ice hockey. Field hockey. Martial arts. Rowing. Canoeing. Kayaking. Surfing. Wrestling.

Sports injury where stretch may be useful
Lower back muscle strain. Lower back ligament sprain. Abdominal muscle strain (obliques).

Additional information for performing this stretch correctly
Keep your thighs vertical, (straight up and down) and your back straight and parallel to the ground. Balance your weight evenly on both your knees and your hand.

Complementary stretch
D23.

D21: STANDING LATERAL SIDE STRETCH

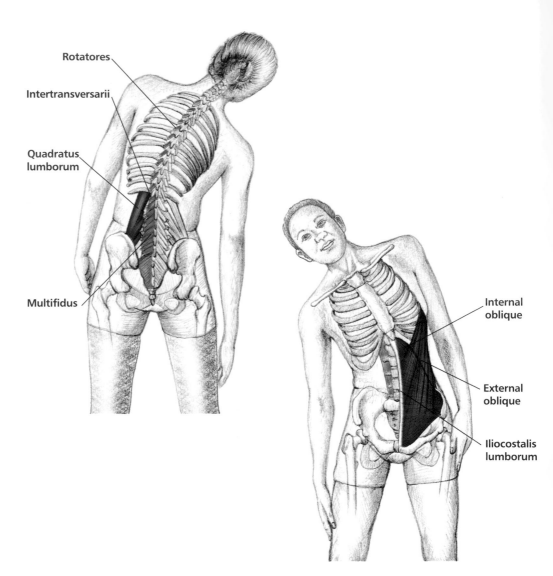

Rotatores

Intertransversarii

Quadratus lumborum

Multifidus

Internal oblique

External oblique

Iliocostalis lumborum

Technique
Stand with your feet about shoulder-width apart and look forward. Keep your body upright and slowly bend to the left or right. Reach down your leg with your hand and do not bend forward.

Muscles being stretched
Primary muscles: Quadratus lumborum. External and internal obliques.
Secondary muscles: Iliocostalis lumborum. Intertransversarii. Rotatores. Multifidus.

Sports that benefit from this stretch
Cricket. Baseball. Softball. Boxing. American football (gridiron). Rugby. Hiking. Backpacking. Mountaineering. Orienteering. Ice hockey. Field hockey. Martial arts. Rowing. Canoeing. Kayaking. Surfing. Wrestling.

Sports injury where stretch may be useful
Lower back muscle strain. Lower back ligament sprain. Abdominal muscle strain (obliques).

Additional information for performing this stretch correctly
Do not lean forward or backward: concentrate on keeping your upper body straight.

Complementary stretch
D23.

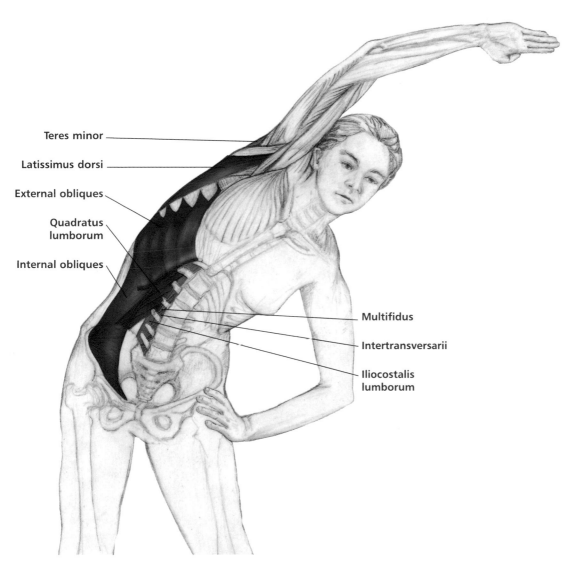

Teres minor

Latissimus dorsi

External obliques

Quadratus lumborum

Internal obliques

Multifidus

Intertransversarii

Iliocostalis lumborum

Technique
Stand with your feet shoulder-width apart, then slowly bend to the side and reach over the top of your head with your hand. Do not bend forward.

Muscles being stretched
Primary muscles: Quadratus lumborum. External and internal obliques. Latissimus dorsi.
Secondary muscles: Teres minor. Iliocostalis lumborum. Intertransversarii. Rotatores. Multifidus.

Sports that benefit from this stretch
Cricket. Baseball. Softball. Boxing. Soccer. American football (gridiron). Rugby. Hiking. Backpacking. Mountaineering. Orienteering. Ice hockey. Field hockey. Martial arts. Rowing. Canoeing. Kayaking. Surfing. Wrestling.

Sports injury where stretch may be useful
Lower back muscle strain. Lower back ligament sprain. Abdominal muscle strain (obliques).

Common problems and more information for performing this stretch correctly
Do not lean forward or backward; concentrate on keeping your upper body straight.

Complementary stretches
D20, D23.

D23: SITTING LATERAL SIDE STRETCH

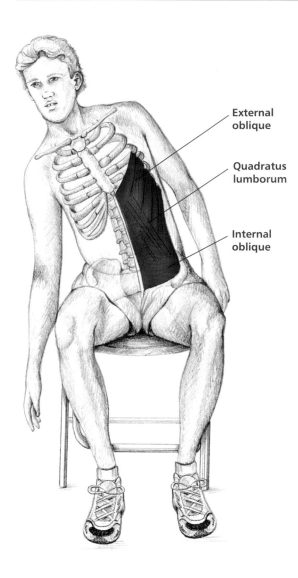

External oblique

Quadratus lumborum

Internal oblique

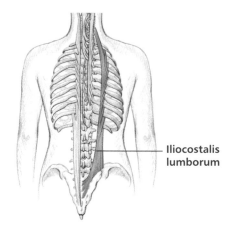

Iliocostalis lumborum

Posterior view.

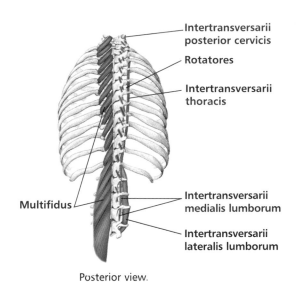

Intertransversarii posterior cervicis

Rotatores

Intertransversarii thoracis

Multifidus

Intertransversarii medialis lumborum

Intertransversarii lateralis lumborum

Posterior view.

Technique
While sitting on a chair with your feet flat on the ground, look straight ahead and keep your body upright. Slowly bend to the left or right while reaching towards the ground with one hand. Do not bend forward.

Muscles being stretched
Primary muscles: Quadratus lumborum. External and internal obliques.
Secondary muscles: Iliocostalis lumborum. Intertransversarii. Rotatores. Multifidus.

Sports that benefit from this stretch
Cricket. Baseball. Softball. Boxing. American football (gridiron). Rugby. Hiking. Backpacking. Mountaineering. Orienteering. Ice hockey. Field hockey. Martial arts. Rowing. Canoeing. Kayaking. Surfing. Wrestling.

Sports injury where stretch may be useful
Lower back muscle strain. Lower back ligament sprain. Abdominal muscle strain (obliques).

Additional information for performing this stretch correctly
Do not lean forward or backward: concentrate on keeping your upper body straight.

Complementary stretch
D06.

7 Hips and Buttocks

The hips and buttocks are comprised of a number of both large muscles (e.g., gluteus maximus) and small muscles (e.g., piriformis). These muscles are primarily responsible for hip stabilisation and lower leg movement. The muscles around the hip and buttocks, along with the structure of the hip joint, allow for a large range of movement of the lower leg; including flexion, extension, adduction, abduction, and rotation.

The **psoas major** runs downwards to be joined by the **iliacus**, together called the *iliopsoas*. Together, these muscles act as padding for various abdominal viscera, and leave the abdomen to become the main flexors of the hip joint, and stabilisers of the low back. Note that some upper fibers of psoas major may insert by a long tendon into the iliopubic eminence to form the **psoas minor**, which has little function and is absent in about 40% of people. Bilateral contracture of this muscle will increase lumbar lordosis.

The bulk of the buttock is mainly formed by the **gluteus maximus**, which is the largest and most superficial muscle of the group, lying posterior to smaller muscles such as gluteus medius and gluteus minimus. Gluteus maximus contributes to powerful hip extension for explosive activities such as sprinting.

Piriformis is a small, tubular muscle that originates at the internal surface of the sacrum, inserts at the superior border of the greater trochanter of the femur, and leaves the pelvis by passing through the greater sciatic foramen. The muscle assists in laterally rotating the hip joint, abducting the thigh when the hip is flexed, and helps to hold the head (ball) of the femur in the *acetabulum* (socket).

The **gemellus superior** and **gemellus inferior** (the *gemelli*) are small, thin muscles that cross the hip joint from the area of the ischium to the greater trochanter of the femur. Their path is almost horizontal across the joint.

Lying between the two gemelli, the **obturator internus** has a broad origin on a part of the pelvis called the *obturator foramen*, along with portions of the lower iliac bone. Besides being an outward rotator, it is a strong stabiliser of the hip.

The **obturator externus** is an ideal rotator of the hip due to its position. It passes from the lower end of the obturator foramen, then behind the neck of the femur to attach to the greater trochanter of the femur on the medial side. Its line of pull allows the head of the femur to roll laterally inside the socket of the pelvis, creating outward, or external rotation.

The most inferior (lowest) deep rotator is the **quadratus femoris**; it is a short muscle running almost horizontal from the upper portion of the ischial tuberosity to the femur.

Sports that benefit from these hip and buttock stretches include: cycling; hiking, backpacking, mountaineering, and orienteering; ice hockey and field hockey; ice-skating, roller-skating and inline skating; martial arts; rowing, canoeing, and kayaking; running, track, and cross-country; running sports like soccer, American football (gridiron), and rugby; snow skiing and water skiing; walking and race walking.

E01: LYING CROSS-OVER KNEE PULL-DOWN STRETCH

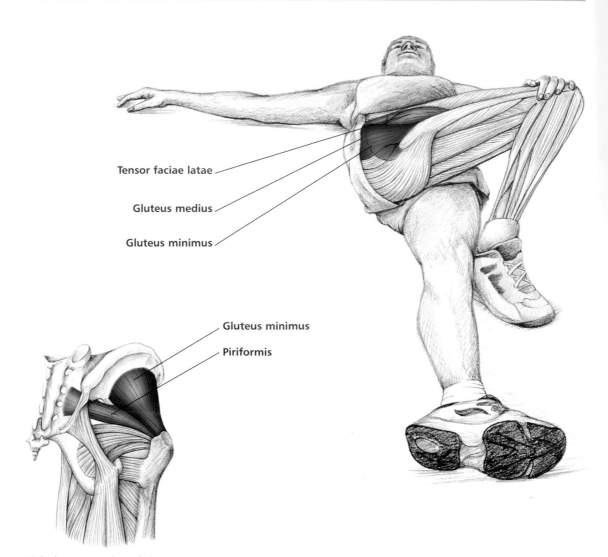

Tensor faciae latae

Gluteus medius

Gluteus minimus

Gluteus minimus

Piriformis

Right leg, posterolateral view.

Technique
Lie on your back and cross one leg over the other. Bring your foot up to your opposite knee and with your opposite arm pull your raised knee towards the ground.

Muscles being stretched
Primary muscles: Gluteus medius and minimus.
Secondary muscles: Tensor fasciae latae. Piriformis.

Sports that benefit from this stretch
Cycling. Hiking. Backpacking. Mountaineering. Orienteering. Ice hockey. Field hockey. Ice-skating. Roller-skating. Inline skating. Martial arts. Running. Track. Cross-country. American football (gridiron). Soccer. Rugby. Snow skiing. Water skiing. Walking. Race walking.

Sports injury where stretch may be useful
Lower back muscle strain. Lower back ligament sprain. Iliotibial band syndrome.

Additional information for performing this stretch correctly
Keep your shoulders on the ground and concentrate on pulling your raised knee to the ground, not up towards your chest.

Complementary stretch
E09.

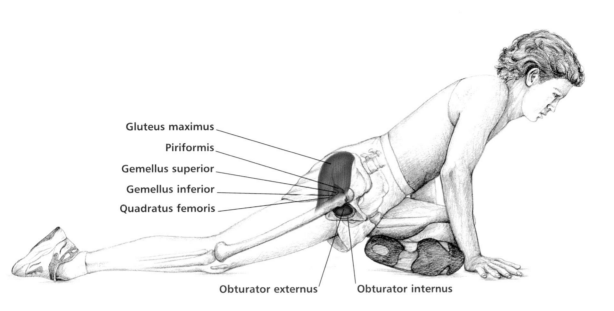

Gluteus maximus
Piriformis
Gemellus superior
Gemellus inferior
Quadratus femoris

Obturator externus   Obturator internus

Technique
Lie on your stomach and bend one leg under your stomach. Lean towards the ground.

Muscles being stretched
Primary muscles: Piriformis. Gemellus superior and inferior. Obturator internus and externus. Quadratus femoris.
Secondary muscle: Gluteus maximus.

Sports that benefit from this stretch
Cycling. Hiking. Backpacking. Mountaineering. Orienteering. Ice hockey. Field hockey. Ice-skating. Roller-skating. Inline skating. Martial arts. Running. Track. Cross-country. American football (gridiron). Soccer. Rugby. Snow skiing. Water skiing. Walking. Race walking.

Sports injury where stretch may be useful
Piriformis syndrome. Snapping hip syndrome. Trochanteric bursitis.

Common problems and additional information for performing this stretch correctly
This position can be a little hard to get into, so make sure you are well supported and use your hands for balance.

Complementary stretch
E04.

E03: STANDING LEG TUCK HIP STRETCH

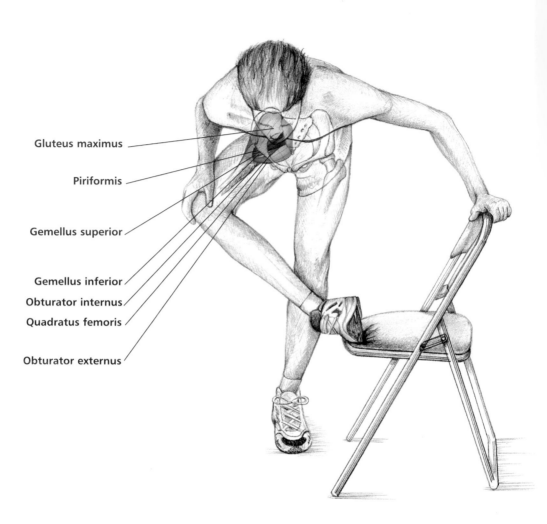

Gluteus maximus

Piriformis

Gemellus superior

Gemellus inferior
Obturator internus
Quadratus femoris

Obturator externus

Technique
Stand beside a chair or table and place the foot furthest from the object onto the object. Relax your leg, lean forward, and bend your other leg, lowering yourself towards the ground.

Muscles being stretched
Primary muscles: Piriformis. Gemellus superior and inferior. Obturator internus and externus. Quadratus femoris.
Secondary muscle: Gluteus maximus.

Sports that benefit from this stretch
Cycling. Hiking. Backpacking. Mountaineering. Orienteering. Ice hockey. Field hockey. Ice-skating. Roller-skating. Inline skating. Martial arts. Running. Track. Cross-country. American football (gridiron). Soccer. Rugby. Snow skiing. Water skiing. Walking. Race walking.

Sports injury where stretch may be useful
Piriformis syndrome. Snapping hip syndrome. Trochanteric bursitis.

Common problems and additional information for performing this stretch correctly
Use the leg you are standing on to regulate the intensity of this stretch. The lower you go, the more tension you will feel.

Complementary stretch
E02.

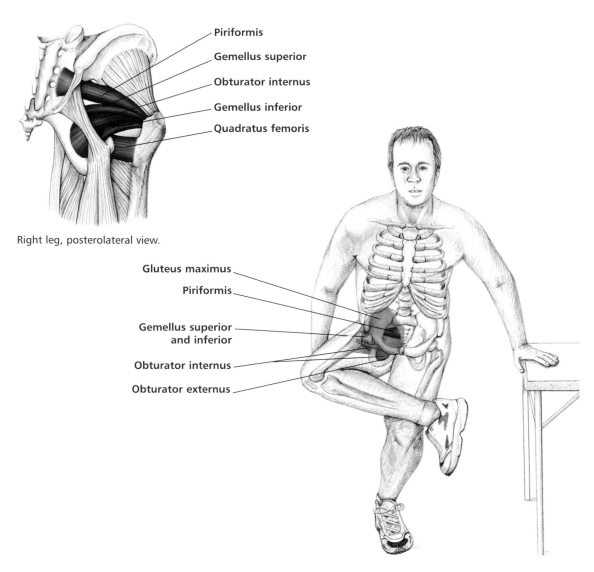

Piriformis
Gemellus superior
Obturator internus
Gemellus inferior
Quadratus femoris

Right leg, posterolateral view.

Gluteus maximus
Piriformis
Gemellus superior and inferior
Obturator internus
Obturator externus

Technique
Stand beside a chair or table for balance, and place one ankle on your opposite knee. Slowly lower yourself towards the ground.

Muscles being stretched
Primary muscles: Piriformis. Gemellus superior and inferior. Obturator internus and externus. Quadratus femoris.
Secondary muscle: Gluteus maximus.

Sports that benefit from this stretch
Cycling. Hiking. Backpacking. Mountaineering. Orienteering. Ice hockey. Field hockey. Ice-skating. Roller-skating. Inline skating. Martial arts. Running. Track. Cross-country. American football (gridiron). Soccer. Rugby. Snow skiing. Water skiing. Walking. Race walking.

Sports injury where stretch may be useful
Piriformis syndrome. Snapping hip syndrome. Trochanteric bursitis.

Common problems and additional information for performing this stretch correctly
Use the leg you are standing on to regulate the intensity of this stretch. The lower you go, the more tension you will feel.

Complementary stretch
E10.

E05: SITTING ROTATIONAL HIP STRETCH

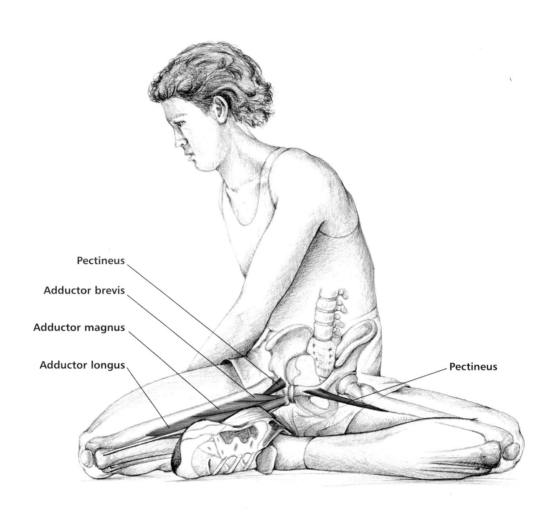

Pectineus

Adductor brevis

Adductor magnus

Adductor longus

Pectineus

Technique
Sit with one leg crossed and your other leg behind your buttocks. Lean your whole body towards the leg that is behind your buttocks.

Muscles being stretched
Primary muscle: Pectineus.
Secondary muscles: Adductor longus, brevis, and magnus.

Sports that benefit from this stretch
Cycling. Hiking. Backpacking. Mountaineering. Orienteering. Ice hockey. Field hockey. Ice-skating. Roller-skating. Inline skating. Martial arts. Running. Track. Cross-country. American football (gridiron). Soccer. Rugby. Snow skiing. Water skiing. Walking. Race walking.

Sports injury where stretch may be useful
Groin strain. Tendonitis of the adductor muscles. Snapping hip syndrome. Trochanteric bursitis.

Additional information for performing this stretch correctly
The more you lean your whole body towards the leg that is behind your buttocks, the more tension you will feel.

Complementary stretch
E06.

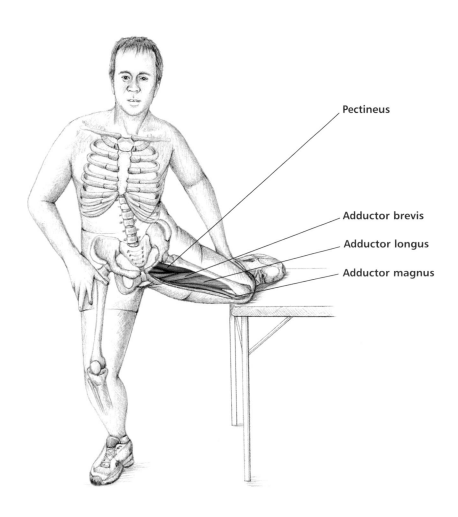

Pectineus

Adductor brevis

Adductor longus

Adductor magnus

Technique
Stand beside a table and raise your lower leg out to the side and up onto the table. Then slowly lower your body.

Muscles being stretched
Primary muscle: Pectineus.
Secondary muscles: Adductor longus, brevis, and magnus.

Sports that benefit from this stretch
Cycling. Hiking. Backpacking. Mountaineering. Orienteering. Ice hockey. Field hockey. Ice-skating. Roller-skating. Inline skating. Martial arts. Running. Track. Cross-country. American football (gridiron). Soccer. Rugby. Snow skiing. Water skiing. Walking. Race walking.

Sports injury where stretch may be useful
Groin strain. Tendonitis of the adductor muscles. Snapping hip syndrome. Trochanteric bursitis.

Common problems and additional information for performing this stretch correctly
Use the leg you are standing on to regulate the intensity of this stretch. The lower you go, the more tension you will feel.

Complementary stretch
E05.

E07: SITTING CROSS-LEGGED REACH FORWARD STRETCH

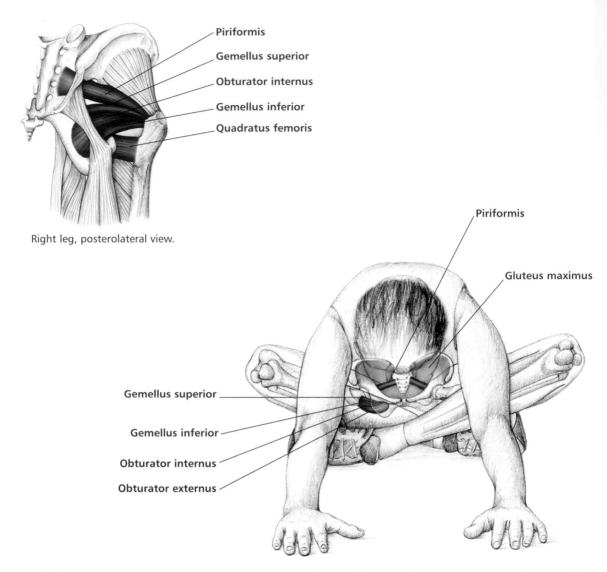

Piriformis
Gemellus superior
Obturator internus
Gemellus inferior
Quadratus femoris

Right leg, posterolateral view.

Piriformis
Gluteus maximus

Gemellus superior
Gemellus inferior
Obturator internus
Obturator externus

Technique
Sit cross-legged and keep your back straight. Then gently lean forward.

Muscles being stretched
Primary muscles: Piriformis. Gemellus superior and inferior. Obturator internus and externus. Quadratus femoris.
Secondary muscle: Gluteus maximus.

Sports that benefit from this stretch
Cycling. Hiking. Backpacking. Mountaineering. Orienteering. Ice hockey. Field hockey. Ice-skating. Roller-skating. Inline skating. Martial arts. Rowing. Canoeing. Kayaking. Running. Track. Cross-country. American football (gridiron). Soccer. Rugby. Snow skiing. Water skiing. Walking. Race walking.

Sports injury where stretch may be useful
Piriformis syndrome. Groin strain. Tendonitis of the adductor muscles. Snapping hip syndrome. Trochanteric bursitis.

Common problems and additional information for performing this stretch correctly
Make the emphasis of this stretch keeping your back straight, rather than trying to lean too far forward.

Complementary stretch
E08.

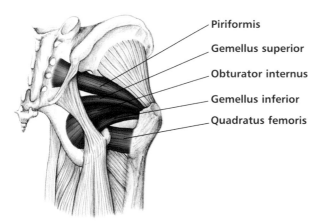

Piriformis
Gemellus superior
Obturator internus
Gemellus inferior
Quadratus femoris

Right leg, posterolateral view.

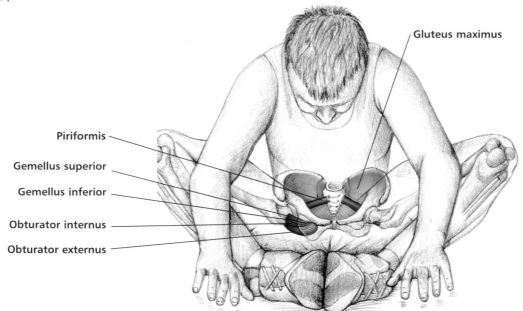

Gluteus maximus

Piriformis
Gemellus superior
Gemellus inferior
Obturator internus
Obturator externus

Technique
Sit with the soles of your feet together and keep your back straight. Then gently lean forward.

Muscles being stretched
Primary muscles: Piriformis. Gemellus superior and inferior. Obturator internus and externus. Quadratus femoris.
Secondary muscle: Gluteus maximus.

Sports that benefit from this stretch
Cycling. Hiking. Backpacking. Mountaineering. Orienteering. Ice hockey. Field hockey. Ice-skating. Roller-skating. Inline skating. Martial arts. Rowing. Canoeing. Kayaking. Running. Track. Cross-country. American football (gridiron). Soccer. Rugby. Snow skiing. Water skiing. Walking. Race walking.

Sports injury where stretch may be useful
Piriformis syndrome. Groin strain. Tendonitis of the adductor muscles. Snapping hip syndrome. Trochanteric bursitis.

Common problems and additional information for performing this stretch correctly
Make the emphasis of this stretch keeping your back straight, rather than trying to lean too far forward.

Complementary stretch
E07.

E09: SITTING KNEE-TO-CHEST BUTTOCKS STRETCH

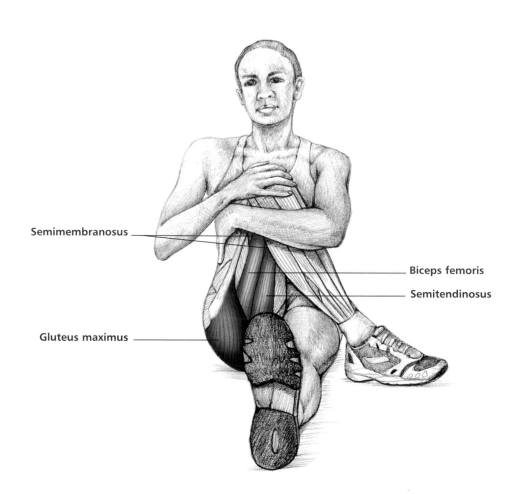

Semimembranosus

Biceps femoris

Semitendinosus

Gluteus maximus

Technique
Sit with one leg straight and the other leg crossed over your knee. Pull the raised knee towards your opposite shoulder while keeping your back straight and your shoulders facing forward.

Muscles being stretched
Primary muscle: Gluteus maximus.
Secondary muscles: Semimembranosus. Semitendinosus. Biceps femoris.

Sports that benefit from this stretch
Cycling. Hiking. Backpacking. Mountaineering. Orienteering. Ice hockey. Field hockey. Ice-skating. Roller-skating. Inline skating. Martial arts. Running. Track. Cross-country. American football (gridiron). Soccer. Rugby. Snow skiing. Water skiing. Walking. Race walking.

Sports injury where stretch may be useful
Lower back muscle strain. Lower back ligament sprain. Hamstring strain. Iliotibial band syndrome.

Common problems and additional information for performing this stretch correctly
Keeping your back straight and your shoulders facing forward will ensure that your buttocks get the maximum benefit from this stretch. Resist the temptation to rotate your shoulders towards your knee.

Complementary stretch
E01.

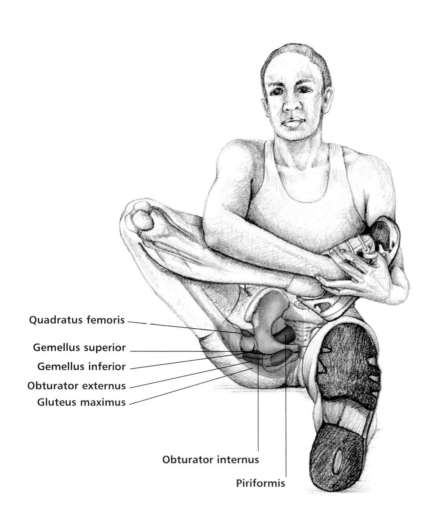

Quadratus femoris

Gemellus superior

Gemellus inferior

Obturator externus

Gluteus maximus

Obturator internus

Piriformis

Technique
Sit with one leg straight and hold onto your other ankle. Pull it directly towards your chest.

Muscles being stretched
Primary muscles: Piriformis. Gemellus superior and inferior. Obturator internus and externus. Quadratus femoris.
Secondary muscle: Gluteus maximus.

Sports that benefit from this stretch
Cycling. Hiking. Backpacking. Mountaineering. Orienteering. Ice hockey. Field hockey. Ice-skating. Roller-skating. Inline skating. Martial arts. Running. Track. Cross-country. American football (gridiron). Soccer. Rugby. Snow skiing. Water skiing. Walking. Race walking.

Sports injury where stretch may be useful
Piriformis syndrome. Snapping hip syndrome. Trochanteric bursitis.

Common problems and additional information for performing this stretch correctly
Use your hands and arms to regulate the intensity of this stretch. The closer you pull your foot to your chest, the more intense the stretch.

Complementary stretch
E04.

E11: LYING CROSS-OVER KNEE PULL-UP STRETCH

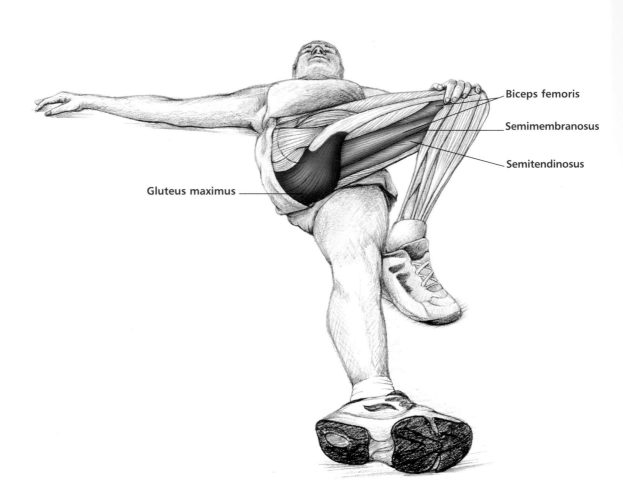

Biceps femoris

Semimembranosus

Semitendinosus

Gluteus maximus

Technique
Lie on your back and cross one leg over the other. Bring your foot up to your opposite knee and with your opposite arm pull your raised knee up towards your chest.

Muscles being stretched
Primary muscle: Gluteus maximus.
Secondary muscles: Semimembranosus. Semitendinosus. Biceps femoris.

Sports that benefit from this stretch
Cycling. Hiking. Backpacking. Mountaineering. Orienteering. Ice hockey. Field hockey. Ice-skating. Roller-skating. Inline skating. Martial arts. Running. Track. Cross-country. American football (gridiron). Soccer. Rugby. Snow skiing. Water skiing. Walking. Race walking.

Sports injury where stretch may be useful
Lower back muscle strain. Lower back ligament sprain. Hamstring strain. Iliotibial band syndrome.

Additional information for performing this stretch correctly
Keep your shoulders on the ground and concentrate on pulling your raised knee up towards your chest, not down towards the ground.

Complementary stretch
E09.

E12: SITTING LEG RESTING BUTTOCKS STRETCH

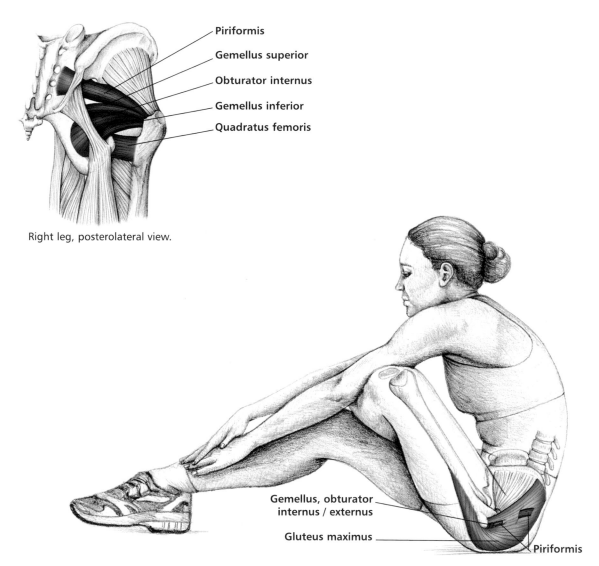

- Piriformis
- Gemellus superior
- Obturator internus
- Gemellus inferior
- Quadratus femoris

Right leg, posterolateral view.

Gemellus, obturator internus / externus
Gluteus maximus
Piriformis

Technique
Sit with one leg slightly bent. Raise the other foot up onto your raised leg and rest it on your thigh, then slowly lean forward.

Muscles being stretched
Primary muscles: Piriformis. Gemellus superior and inferior. Obturator internus and externus. Quadratus femoris.
Secondary muscle: Gluteus maximus.

Sports that benefit from this stretch
Cycling. Hiking. Backpacking. Mountaineering. Orienteering. Ice hockey. Field hockey. Ice-skating. Roller-skating. Inline skating. Martial arts. Running. Track. Cross-country. American football (gridiron). Soccer. Rugby. Snow skiing. Water skiing. Walking. Race walking.

Sports injury where stretch may be useful
Piriformis syndrome. Snapping hip syndrome. Trochanteric bursitis.

Common problems and additional information for performing this stretch correctly
This position can be a little hard to get into, so make sure that you are well supported and use your hands for balance if you need to. To increase the intensity of this stretch, straighten your back and lean forward.

Complementary stretch
E10.

E13: LYING LEG RESTING BUTTOCKS STRETCH

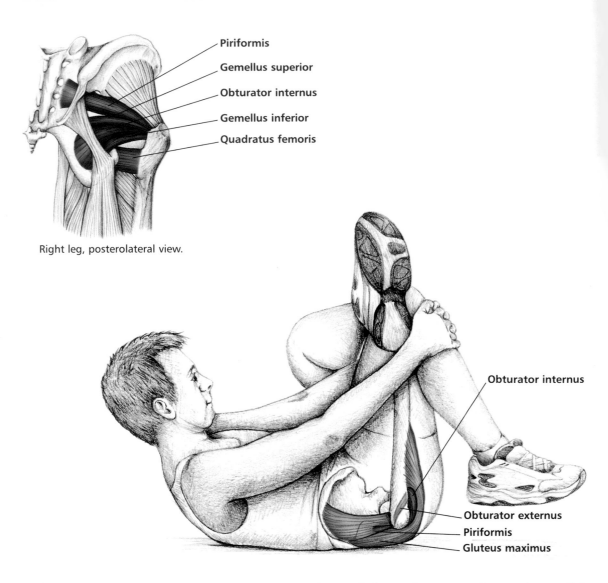

Piriformis
Gemellus superior
Obturator internus
Gemellus inferior
Quadratus femoris

Right leg, posterolateral view.

Obturator internus
Obturator externus
Piriformis
Gluteus maximus

Technique
Lie on your back and slightly bend one leg. Raise the other foot up onto your bent leg and rest it on your thigh. Then reach forward, holding onto your knee and pull it towards you.

Muscles being stretched
Primary muscles: Piriformis. Gemellus superior and inferior. Obturator internus and externus. Quadratus femoris.
Secondary muscle: Gluteus maximus.

Sports that benefit from this stretch
Cycling. Hiking. Backpacking. Mountaineering. Orienteering. Ice hockey. Field hockey. Ice-skating. Roller-skating. Inline skating. Martial arts. Running. Track. Cross-country. American football (gridiron). Soccer. Rugby. Snow skiing. Water skiing. Walking. Race walking.

Sports injury where stretch may be useful
Piriformis syndrome. Snapping hip syndrome. Trochanteric bursitis.

Additional information for performing this stretch correctly
Regulate the intensity of this stretch by pulling your knee towards you.

Complementary stretch
E12.

8 Quadriceps

The quadriceps is a large group of muscles, the most massive of the leg, located in the anterior (front) of the thigh. They originate from above the hip joint and extend to below the knee. The primary action of the quadriceps is to extend the knee joint, but in conjunction with a number of other muscles in the front of the hip, they are also associated with hip flexion.

Rectus femoris is part of the quadriceps femoris, which also includes the vasti group: **vastus lateralis**, **vastus medialis**, and **vastus intermedius**. It has two heads of origin. The reflected head is in the line of pull of the muscle in four-footed animals, whereas the straight head seems to have developed in humans as a result of the upright posture. It is a spindle shaped bi-pennate muscle.

The quadriceps straighten the knee when rising from sitting, during walking, and climbing. The vasti muscles cross only the knee, and thus are limited to knee extension or resistance to knee flexion; they spread out to control the movement of sitting down. Vastus medialis is larger and heavier than vastus lateralis. Vastus intermedius is the deepest part of the quadriceps femoris, and has a membranous tendon on its anterior surface to allow a gliding movement between itself and the rectus femoris that overlies it. The quadriceps tendon attaches to, and covers the patella, becoming the patellar tendon below this and attaching to the tibia.

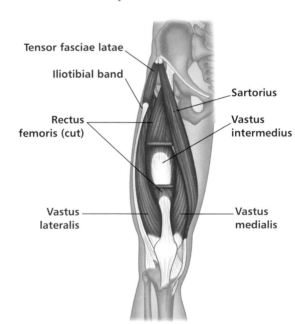

Tensor fasciae latae

Iliotibial band

Rectus femoris (cut)

Vastus lateralis

Sartorius

Vastus intermedius

Vastus medialis

Included here is **sartorius**, not part of the quadriceps femoris group, but the most superficial muscle of the anterior thigh; it is also the longest strap muscle in the body. The medial border of the upper third of this muscle forms the lateral boundary of the femoral triangle (adductor longus forms the medial boundary; the inguinal ligament forms the superior boundary). The action of sartorius is to put the lower limbs in the cross-legged seated position of the tailor (hence its name from the Latin).

Sports that benefit from these quadriceps stretches include: cycling; hiking, backpacking, mountaineering, and orienteering; ice hockey and field hockey; ice-skating, roller-skating, and inline skating; martial arts; running, track, and cross-country; running sports like soccer, American football (gridiron), and rugby; snow skiing and water skiing; surfing; walking and race walking.

F01: KNEELING QUAD STRETCH

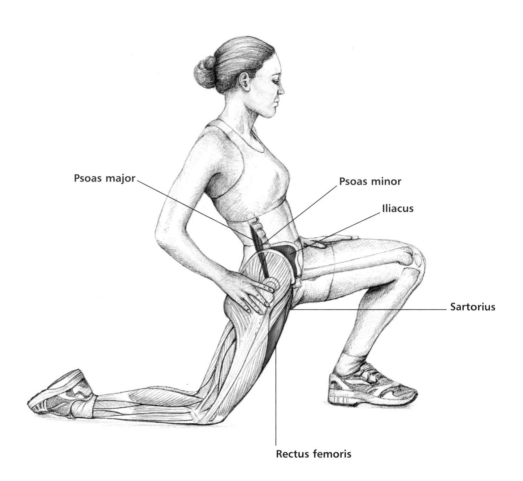

Psoas major

Psoas minor

Iliacus

Sartorius

Rectus femoris

Technique
Kneel on one foot and the other knee. If needed, hold on to something to keep your balance. Push your hips forward.

Muscles being stretched
Primary muscles: Iliacus. Psoas major and minor.
Secondary muscles: Rectus femoris. Sartorius.

Sports that benefit from this stretch
Cycling. Hiking. Backpacking. Mountaineering. Orienteering. Ice hockey. Field hockey. Ice-skating. Roller-skating. Inline skating. Martial arts. Running. Track. Cross-country. American football (gridiron). Soccer. Rugby. Snow skiing. Water skiing. Surfing. Walking. Race walking.

Sports injury where stretch may be useful
Hip flexor strain. Avulsion fracture in the pelvic area. Osteitis pubis. Iliopsoas tendonitis. Trochanteric bursitis. Quadriceps strain. Quadriceps tendonitis.

Common problems and more information for performing this stretch correctly
Regulate the intensity of this stretch by pushing your hips forward. If need be, place a towel or mat under your knee for comfort.

Complementary stretch
F05.

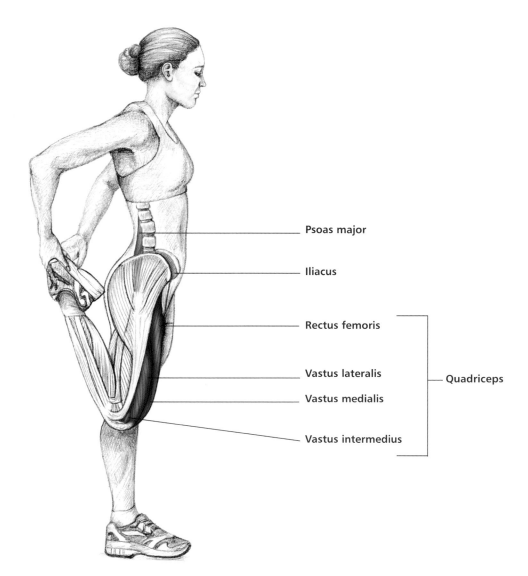

Psoas major

Iliacus

Rectus femoris

Vastus lateralis

Vastus medialis

Vastus intermedius

Quadriceps

Technique
Stand upright while balancing on one leg. Pull your other foot up behind your buttocks and keep your knees together while pushing your hips forward. Hold on to something for balance.

Muscles being stretched
Primary muscles: Rectus femoris. Vastus medialis, lateralis, and intermedius. Secondary muscles: Iliacus. Psoas major.

Sports that benefit from this stretch
Cycling. Hiking. Backpacking. Mountaineering. Orienteering. Ice hockey. Field hockey. Ice-skating. Roller-skating. Inline skating. Martial arts. Running. Track. Cross-country. American football (gridiron). Soccer. Rugby. Snow skiing. Water skiing. Surfing. Walking. Race walking.

Sports injury where stretch may be useful
Hip flexor strain. Avulsion fracture in the pelvic area. Osteitis pubis. Iliopsoas tendonitis. Trochanteric bursitis. Quadriceps strain. Quadriceps tendonitis. Patellofemoral pain syndrome. Patellar tendonitis. Subluxing kneecap.

Common problems and more information for performing this stretch correctly
This position can put undue pressure on the knee joint and ligaments. Anyone with knee pain or knee injury should avoid this stretch.

Complementary stretch
F04.

F03: STANDING REACH-UP QUAD STRETCH

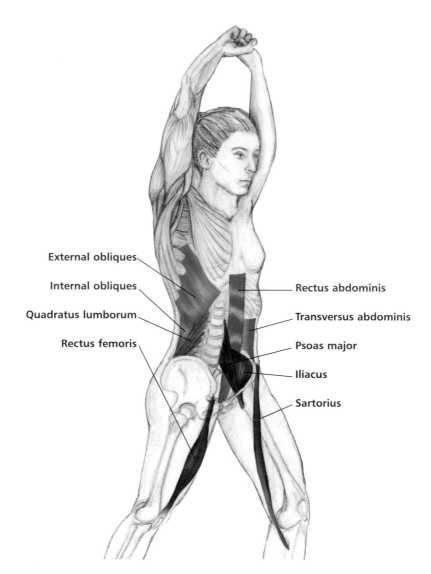

External obliques

Internal obliques

Quadratus lumborum

Rectus femoris

Rectus abdominis

Transversus abdominis

Psoas major

Iliacus

Sartorius

Technique
Stand upright and take one small step forward. Reach up with both hands, push your hips forward, lean back, and then lean away from your back leg.

Muscles being stretched
Primary muscles: Rectus femoris. Psoas major. Iliacus. Sartorius.
Secondary muscles: Rectus abdominis. Transversus abdominis. External and internal obliques. Quadratus lumborum.

Sports that benefit from this stretch
Cycling. Hiking. Backpacking. Mountaineering. Orienteering. Ice hockey. Field hockey. Ice-skating. Roller-skating. Inline skating. Martial arts. Running. Track. Cross-country. Soccer. American football (gridiron). Rugby. Snow skiing. Water skiing. Surfing. Walking. Race walking.

Sports injury where stretch may be useful
Hip flexor strain. Avulsion fracture in the pelvic area. Osteitis pubis. Iliopsoas tendonitis. Trochanteric bursitis. Quadriceps strain. Quadriceps tendonitis.

Additional information for performing this stretch correctly
Regulate the intensity of this stretch by pushing your hips forward.

Complementary stretches
F01, C03.

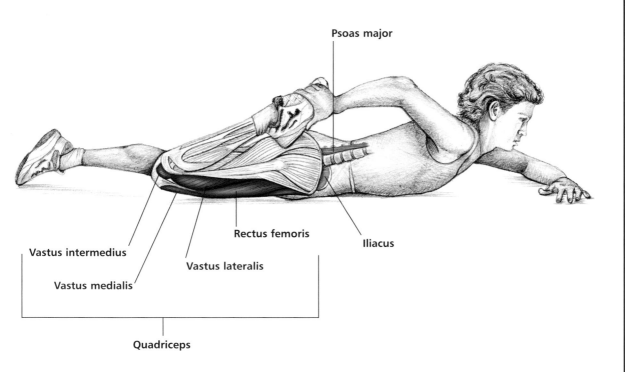

Psoas major

Rectus femoris

Iliacus

Vastus intermedius

Vastus lateralis

Vastus medialis

Quadriceps

Technique
Lie face down and pull one foot up behind your buttocks.

Muscles being stretched
Primary muscles: Rectus femoris. Vastus medialis, lateralis, and intermedius. Secondary muscles: Iliacus. Psoas major.

Sports that benefit from this stretch
Cycling. Hiking. Backpacking. Mountaineering. Orienteering. Ice hockey. Field hockey. Ice-skating. Roller-skating. Inline skating. Martial arts. Running. Track. Cross-country. American football (gridiron). Soccer. Rugby. Snow skiing. Water skiing. Surfing. Walking. Race walking.

Sports injury where stretch may be useful
Hip flexor strain. Avulsion fracture in the pelvic area. Osteitis pubis. Iliopsoas tendonitis. Trochanteric bursitis. Quadriceps strain. Quadriceps tendonitis. Patellofemoral pain syndrome. Patellar tendonitis. Subluxing kneecap.

Common problems and more information for performing this stretch correctly
This position can put undue pressure on the knee joint and ligaments. Anyone with knee pain or knee injury should avoid this stretch.

Complementary stretch
F02.

F05: ON-YOUR-SIDE QUAD STRETCH

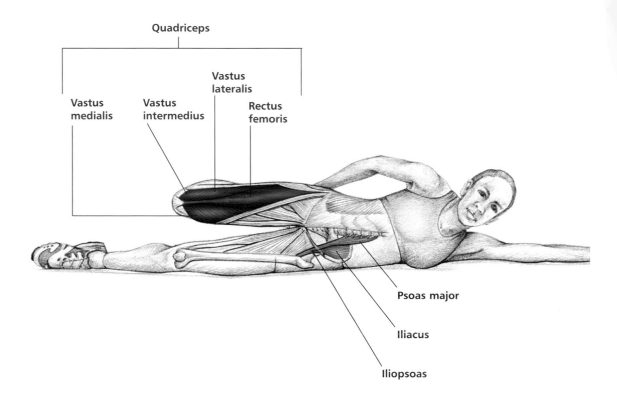

Quadriceps

Vastus lateralis

Vastus medialis

Vastus intermedius

Rectus femoris

Psoas major

Iliacus

Iliopsoas

Technique
Lie on your side and pull your top leg behind your buttocks. Keep your knees together and push your hips forward.

Muscles being stretched
Primary muscles: Rectus femoris. Vastus medialis, lateralis, and intermedius. Secondary muscles: Iliacus. Psoas major.

Sports that benefit from this stretch
Cycling. Hiking. Backpacking. Mountaineering. Orienteering. Ice hockey. Field hockey. Ice-skating. Roller-skating. Inline skating. Martial arts. Running. Track. Cross-country. American football (gridiron). Soccer. Rugby. Snow skiing. Water skiing. Surfing. Walking. Race walking.

Sports injury where stretch may be useful
Hip flexor strain. Avulsion fracture in the pelvic area. Osteitis pubis. Iliopsoas tendonitis. Trochanteric bursitis. Quadriceps strain. Quadriceps tendonitis. Patellofemoral pain syndrome. Patellar tendonitis. Subluxing kneecap.

Common problems and more information for performing this stretch correctly
This position can put undue pressure on the knee joint and ligaments. Anyone with knee pain or knee injury should avoid this stretch.

Complementary stretch
F01.

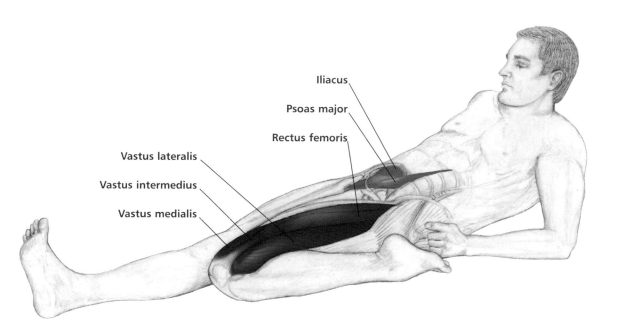

Iliacus

Psoas major

Rectus femoris

Vastus lateralis

Vastus intermedius

Vastus medialis

Technique
Sit on the ground, bend one knee and place that foot next to your buttocks. Then slowly lean backwards.

Muscles being stretched
Primary muscles: Rectus femoris. Vastus medialis, lateralis, and intermedius.
Secondary muscles: Iliacus. Psoas major.

Sports that benefit from this stretch
Cycling. Hiking. Backpacking. Mountaineering. Orienteering. Ice hockey. Field hockey. Ice-skating. Roller-skating. Inline skating. Martial arts. Running. Track. Cross-country. Soccer. American football (gridiron). Rugby. Snow skiing. Water skiing. Surfing. Walking. Race walking.

Sports injury where stretch may be useful
Hip flexor strain. Avulsion fracture in the pelvic area. Osteitis pubis. Iliopsoas tendonitis. Trochanteric bursitis. Quadriceps strain. Quadriceps tendonitis. Patellofemoral pain syndrome. Patellar tendonitis. Subluxing kneecap.

Common problems and more information for performing this stretch correctly
This position can put undue pressure on the knee joint and ligaments. Anyone with knee pain or knee injury should avoid this stretch.

Complementary stretches
F05, C03.

F07: DOUBLE LEAN-BACK QUAD STRETCH

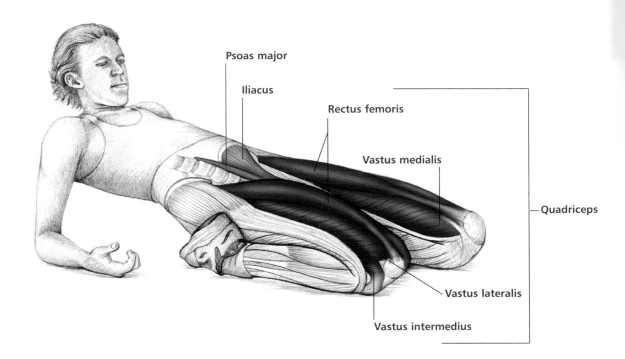

Psoas major

Iliacus

Rectus femoris

Vastus medialis

Quadriceps

Vastus lateralis

Vastus intermedius

Technique
Sit on the ground and bend one or both knees and place your legs under your buttocks. Then slowly lean backwards.

Muscles being stretched
Primary muscles: Rectus femoris. Vastus medialis, lateralis, and intermedius. Secondary muscles: Iliacus. Psoas major.

Sports that benefit from this stretch
Cycling. Hiking. Backpacking. Mountaineering. Orienteering. Ice hockey. Field hockey. Ice-skating. Roller-skating. Inline skating. Martial arts. Running. Track. Cross-country. American football (gridiron). Soccer. Rugby. Snow skiing. Water skiing. Surfing. Walking. Race walking.

Sports injury where stretch may be useful
Hip flexor strain. Avulsion fracture in the pelvic area. Osteitis pubis. Iliopsoas tendonitis. Trochanteric bursitis. Quadriceps strain. Quadriceps tendonitis. Patellofemoral pain syndrome. Patellar tendonitis. Subluxing kneecap.

Common problems and more information for performing this stretch correctly
This position can put undue pressure on the knee joint and ligaments. Anyone with knee pain or knee injury should avoid this stretch.

Complementary stretch
F02.

The hamstrings are a large group of three separate muscles located in the posterior (rear) of the thigh. They originate from the bottom of the hip bone and extend to below the knee, and work together to extend the hip and flex the knee; they correspond to the flexors of the elbow in the upper limb. During running, the hamstrings slow down the leg at the end of its forward swing and prevent the trunk from flexing at the hip joint. The three muscles are, from medial to lateral, **semimembranosus**, **semitendinosus**, and **biceps femoris**. Biceps femoris is usually the largest hamstring, and has two heads, the long and short; the long head crosses the hip joint to work it. Semitendinosus and semimembranosus are completely synergistic, meaning they both do the exact same actions.

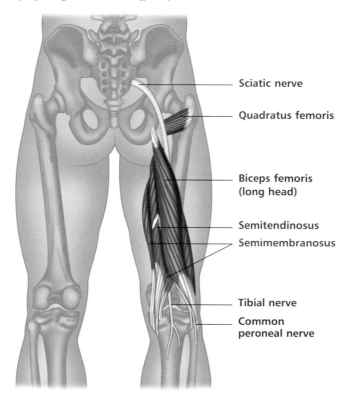

Sciatic nerve

Quadratus femoris

Biceps femoris (long head)

Semitendinosus

Semimembranosus

Tibial nerve

Common peroneal nerve

Sports that benefit from these hamstring stretches include: basketball and netball; cycling; hiking, backpacking, mountaineering, and orienteering; ice hockey and field hockey; ice-skating, roller-skating, and inline skating; martial arts; running, track, and cross-country; running sports like soccer, American football (gridiron), and rugby; snow skiing and water skiing; surfing; walking and race walking; wrestling.

G01: SITTING REACH FORWARD HAMSTRING STRETCH

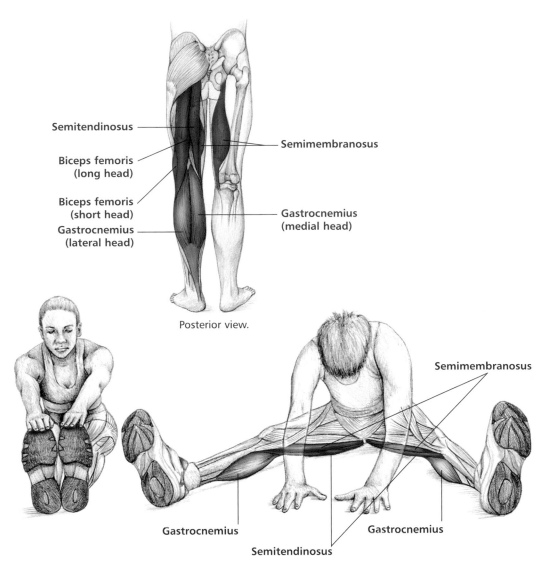

Semitendinosus

Biceps femoris
(long head)

Biceps femoris
(short head)

Gastrocnemius
(lateral head)

Semimembranosus

Gastrocnemius
(medial head)

Posterior view.

Semimembranosus

Gastrocnemius

Gastrocnemius

Semitendinosus

Technique
Sit with both legs straight out in front and keep your toes pointing straight up. Make sure your back is straight and then reach forward towards your toes.

Muscles being stretched
Primary muscles: Semimembranosus. Semitendinosus. Biceps femoris. Secondary muscle: Gastrocnemius.

Sports that benefit from this stretch
Basketball. Netball. Cycling. Hiking. Backpacking. Mountaineering. Orienteering. Ice hockey. Field hockey. Ice-skating. Roller-skating. Inline skating. Martial arts. Running. Track. Cross-country. American football (gridiron). Soccer. Rugby. Snow skiing. Water skiing. Surfing. Walking. Race walking. Wrestling.

Sports injury where stretch may be useful
Lower back muscle strain. Lower back ligament sprain. Hamstring strain.

Common problems and additional information for performing this stretch correctly
It is important to keep your toes pointing straight upwards. Letting your toes fall to one side will cause this stretch to put uneven tension on the hamstring muscles. Over an extended period of time, this could lead to a muscle imbalance.

Complementary stretch
G06.

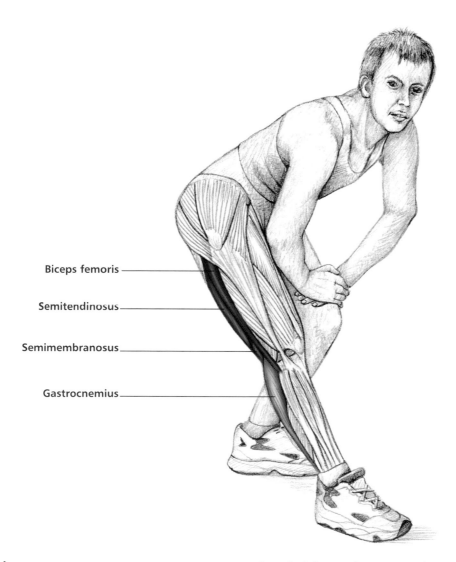

Biceps femoris

Semitendinosus

Semimembranosus

Gastrocnemius

Technique
Stand with one knee bent and the other leg straight out in front. Point your toes towards the ground and lean forward. Keep your back straight and rest your hands on your bent knee.

Muscles being stretched
Primary muscles: Semimembranosus. Semitendinosus. Biceps femoris. Secondary muscle: Gastrocnemius.

Sports that benefit from this stretch
Basketball. Netball. Cycling. Hiking. Backpacking. Mountaineering. Orienteering. Ice hockey. Field hockey. Ice-skating. Roller-skating. Inline skating. Martial arts. Running. Track. Cross-country. American football (gridiron). Soccer. Rugby. Snow skiing. Water skiing. Surfing. Walking. Race walking. Wrestling.

Sports injury where stretch may be useful
Lower back muscle strain. Lower back ligament sprain. Hamstring strain.

Additional information for performing this stretch correctly
Regulate the intensity of this stretch by keeping your back straight and leaning forward.

Complementary stretch
G03.

G03: STANDING TOE-RAISED HAMSTRING STRETCH

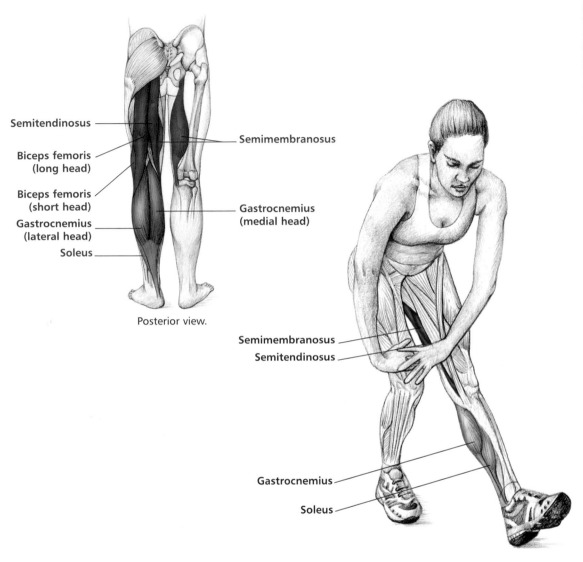

Semitendinosus

Biceps femoris (long head)

Biceps femoris (short head)

Gastrocnemius (lateral head)

Soleus

Semimembranosus

Gastrocnemius (medial head)

Posterior view.

Semimembranosus
Semitendinosus

Gastrocnemius

Soleus

Technique
Stand with one knee bent and the other leg straight out in front. Point your toes towards your body and lean forward. Keep your back straight and rest your hands on your bent knee.

Muscles being stretched
Primary muscles: Semimembranosus. Semitendinosus. Biceps femoris. Secondary muscles: Gastrocnemius. Soleus.

Sports that benefit from this stretch
Basketball. Netball. Cycling. Hiking. Backpacking. Mountaineering. Orienteering. Ice hockey. Field hockey. Ice-skating. Roller-skating. Inline skating. Martial arts. Running. Track. Cross-country. American football (gridiron). Soccer. Rugby. Snow skiing. Water skiing. Surfing. Walking. Race walking. Wrestling.

Sports injury where stretch may be useful
Lower back muscle strain. Lower back ligament sprain. Hamstring strain. Calf strain.

Additional information for performing this stretch correctly
Regulate the intensity of this stretch by keeping your back straight and flexing your ankle so that your toes are pointing upwards.

Complementary stretch
G04.

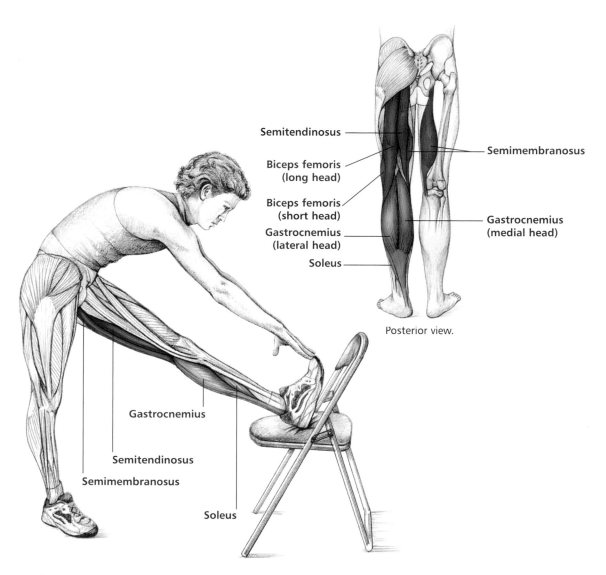

Semitendinosus

Biceps femoris
(long head)

Biceps femoris
(short head)

Gastrocnemius
(lateral head)

Soleus

Semimembranosus

Gastrocnemius
(medial head)

Posterior view.

Gastrocnemius

Semitendinosus

Semimembranosus

Soleus

Technique
Stand upright and raise one leg on to an object.
Keep that leg straight and your toes pointing
straight up. Lean forward while keeping your
back straight.

Muscles being stretched
Primary muscles: Semimembranosus.
Semitendinosus. Biceps femoris.
Secondary muscles: Gastrocnemius. Soleus.

Sports that benefit from this stretch
Basketball. Netball. Cycling. Hiking. Backpacking.
Mountaineering. Orienteering. Ice hockey. Field
hockey. Ice-skating. Roller-skating. Inline skating.
Martial arts. Running. Track. Cross-country.
American football (gridiron). Soccer. Rugby. Snow
skiing. Water skiing. Surfing. Walking. Race
walking. Wrestling.

Sports injury where stretch may be useful
Lower back muscle strain. Lower back ligament
sprain. Hamstring strain. Calf strain.

Common problems and additional information for performing this stretch correctly
Regulate the intensity of this stretch by keeping
your back straight and leaning forward.

Complementary stretch
G01.

G05: STANDING LEG-UP TOE-IN HAMSTRING STRETCH

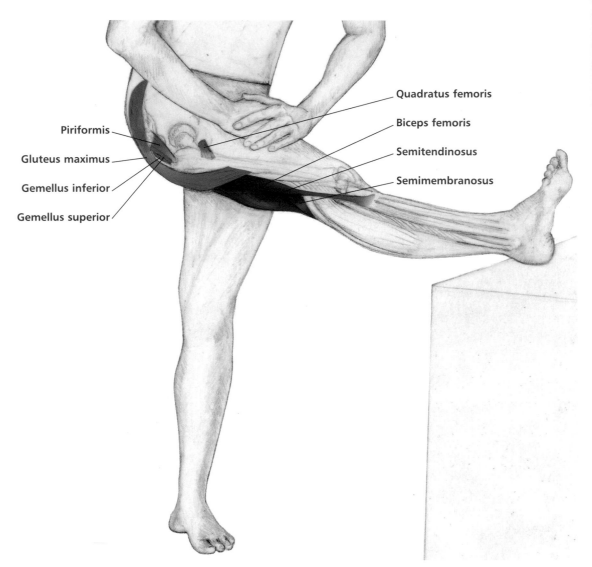

Piriformis

Gluteus maximus

Gemellus inferior

Gemellus superior

Quadratus femoris

Biceps femoris

Semitendinosus

Semimembranosus

Technique
Stand upright and raise one leg on to an object. Keep that leg straight and point your toes upwards. Then turn the other foot inward and lean forward whilst keeping your back straight.

Muscles being stretched
Primary muscles: Semimembranosus. Semitendinosus. Biceps femoris. Secondary muscles: Gluteus maximus. Gemellus inferior and superior. Quadratus femoris. Piriformis.

Sports that benefit from this stretch
Basketball. Netball. Cycling. Hiking. Backpacking. Mountaineering. Orienteering. Ice hockey. Field hockey. Ice-skating. Roller-skating. Inline skating. Martial arts. Running. Track. Cross-country. Soccer. American football (gridiron). Rugby. Snow skiing. Water skiing. Surfing. Walking. Race walking. Wrestling.

Sports injury where stretch may be useful
Lower back muscle strain. Lower back ligament sprain. Hamstring strain. Calf strain.

Common problems and more information for performing this stretch correctly
This stretch can put intense pressure on the deep lateral hip rotators. Regulate the intensity of this stretch by keeping your back straight and slowly leaning forward.

Complementary stretches
G11, E01.

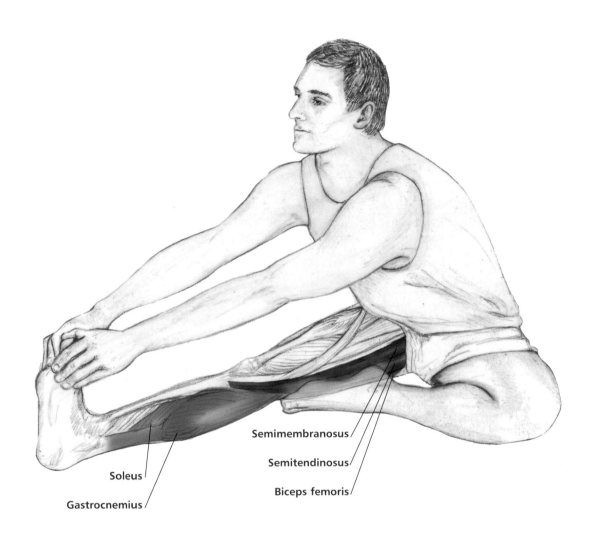

Semimembranosus

Semitendinosus

Biceps femoris

Soleus

Gastrocnemius

Technique
Sit with one leg straight out in front and toes pointing upwards. Bring your other foot towards your knee. Reach toward your toes with both hands.

Muscles being stretched
Primary muscles: Semimembranosus. Semitendinosus. Biceps femoris. Secondary muscles: Gastrocnemius. Soleus.

Sports that benefit from this stretch
Basketball. Netball. Cycling. Hiking. Backpacking. Mountaineering. Orienteering. Ice hockey. Field hockey. Ice-skating. Roller-skating. Inline skating. Martial arts. Running. Track. Cross-country. American football (gridiron). Soccer. Rugby. Snow skiing. Water skiing. Surfing. Walking. Race walking. Wrestling.

Sports injury where stretch may be useful
Lower back muscle strain. Lower back ligament sprain. Hamstring strain. Calf strain.

Common problems and additional information for performing this stretch correctly
It is important to keep your toes pointing straight upwards. Letting your toes fall to one side will cause this stretch to put uneven tension on the hamstring muscles. Over an extended period of time, this could lead to a muscle imbalance.

Complementary stretch
G09.

G07: LYING PARTNER ASSISTED HAMSTRING STRETCH

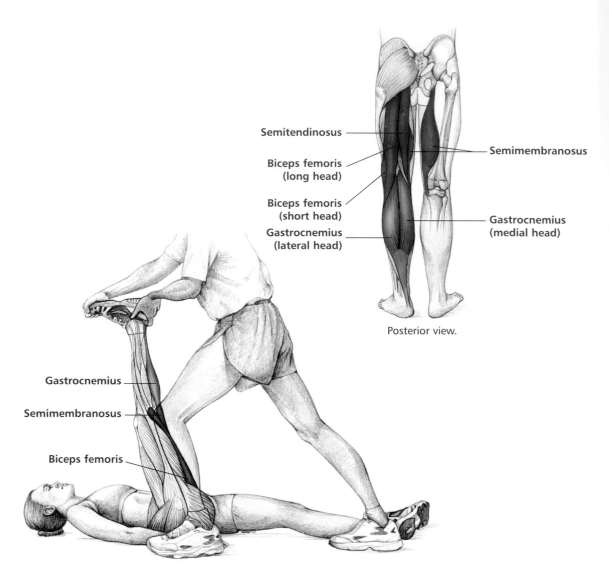

Semitendinosus

Biceps femoris (long head)

Biceps femoris (short head)

Gastrocnemius (lateral head)

Semimembranosus

Gastrocnemius (medial head)

Posterior view.

Gastrocnemius

Semimembranosus

Biceps femoris

Technique
Lie on your back and keep both legs straight. Have a partner raise one of your legs off the ground and as far back as is comfortable. Make sure your toes are pointing directly backwards.

Muscles being stretched
Primary muscles: Semimembranosus. Semitendinosus. Biceps femoris. Secondary muscle: Gastrocnemius.

Sports that benefit from this stretch
Basketball. Netball. Cycling. Hiking. Backpacking. Mountaineering. Orienteering. Ice hockey. Field hockey. Ice-skating. Roller-skating. Inline skating. Martial arts. Running. Track. Cross-country. American football (gridiron). Soccer. Rugby. Snow skiing. Water skiing. Surfing. Walking. Race walking. Wrestling.

Sports injury where stretch may be useful
Lower back muscle strain. Lower back ligament sprain. Hamstring strain. Calf strain.

Common problems and additional information for performing this stretch correctly
Choose your stretching partner carefully. They are responsible for your safety while performing this stretch, so make sure you communicate clearly with them at all times.

Complementary stretch
G04.

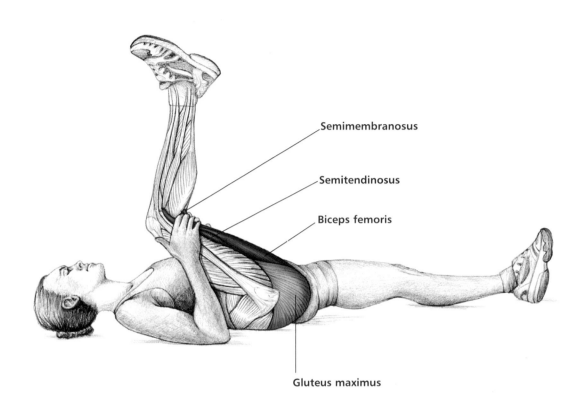

Semimembranosus

Semitendinosus

Biceps femoris

Gluteus maximus

Technique
Lie on your back and bend one leg. Pull the other knee towards your chest, then slowly and gently straighten your raised leg.

Muscles being stretched
Primary muscles: Semimembranosus. Semitendinosus. Biceps femoris. Secondary muscle: Gluteus maximus.

Sports that benefit from this stretch
Basketball. Netball. Cycling. Hiking. Backpacking. Mountaineering. Orienteering. Ice hockey. Field hockey. Ice-skating. Roller-skating. Inline skating. Martial arts. Running. Track. Cross-country. American football (gridiron). Soccer. Rugby. Snow skiing. Water skiing. Surfing. Walking. Race walking. Wrestling.

Sports injury where stretch may be useful
Lower back muscle strain. Lower back ligament sprain. Hamstring strain.

Additional information for performing this stretch correctly
Keep your upper leg (thigh) relatively still, and regulate the intensity of this stretch by straightening your knee.

Complementary stretch
G12.

G09: LYING STRAIGHT KNEE HAMSTRING STRETCH

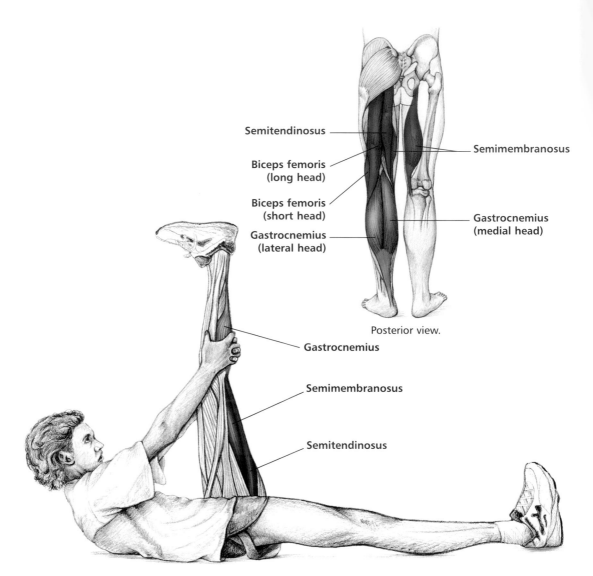

Semitendinosus

Semimembranosus

Biceps femoris (long head)

Biceps femoris (short head)

Gastrocnemius (medial head)

Gastrocnemius (lateral head)

Posterior view.

Gastrocnemius

Semimembranosus

Semitendinosus

Technique
Lie on your back and bend one leg. Raise your straight leg and pull it towards your chest.

Muscles being stretched
Primary muscles: Semimembranosus. Semitendinosus. Biceps femoris. Secondary muscle: Gastrocnemius.

Sports that benefit from this stretch
Basketball. Netball. Cycling. Hiking. Backpacking. Mountaineering. Orienteering. Ice hockey. Field hockey. Ice-skating. Roller-skating. Inline skating. Martial arts. Running. Track. Cross-country. American football (gridiron). Soccer. Rugby. Snow skiing. Water skiing. Surfing. Walking. Race walking. Wrestling.

Sports injury where stretch may be useful
Lower back muscle strain. Lower back ligament sprain. Hamstring strain. Calf strain.

Common problems and additional information for performing this stretch correctly
It is important to keep your toes pointing straight backwards. Letting your toes fall to one side will cause this stretch to put uneven tension on the hamstring muscles. Over an extended period of time, this could lead to a muscle imbalance.

Complementary stretch
G10.

G10: KNEELING TOE-RAISED HAMSTRING STRETCH

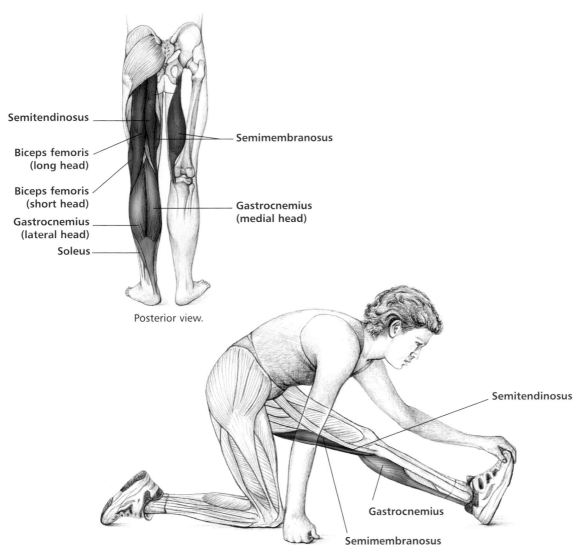

Semitendinosus

Semimembranosus

Biceps femoris (long head)

Biceps femoris (short head)

Gastrocnemius (medial head)

Gastrocnemius (lateral head)

Soleus

Posterior view.

Semitendinosus

Gastrocnemius

Semimembranosus

Technique
Kneel on one knee and place your other leg forward with your heel on the ground. Keep your back straight and point your toes towards your body. Reach towards your toes with one hand.

Muscles being stretched
Primary muscles: Semimembranosus. Semitendinosus. Biceps femoris. Secondary muscle: Gastrocnemius. Soleus.

Sports that benefit from this stretch
Basketball. Netball. Cycling. Hiking. Backpacking. Mountaineering. Orienteering. Ice hockey. Field hockey. Ice-skating. Roller-skating. Inline skating. Martial arts. Running. Track. Cross-country. American football (gridiron). Soccer. Rugby. Snow skiing. Water skiing. Surfing. Walking. Race walking. Wrestling.

Sports injury where stretch may be useful
Lower back muscle strain. Lower back ligament sprain. Hamstring strain. Calf strain.

Common problems and additional information for performing this stretch correctly
It is not important to be able to touch your toes. Concentrate on keeping your back straight and your toes pointing up.

Complementary stretch
G03.

G11: SITTING LEG RESTING HAMSTRING STRETCH

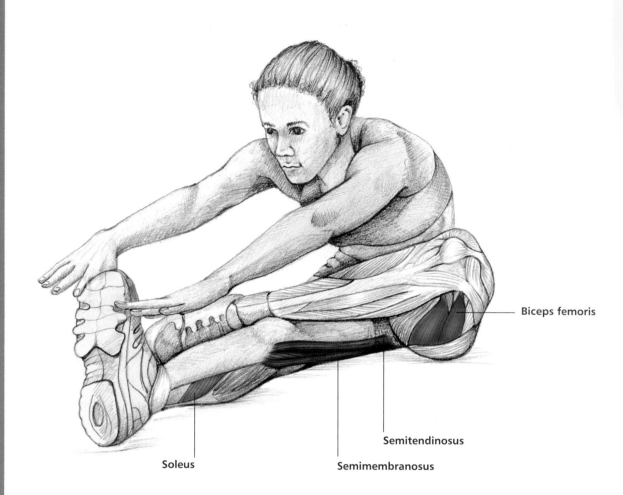

Biceps femoris

Semitendinosus

Semimembranosus

Soleus

Technique
Sit with one leg straight out in front and keep your toes pointing up. Cross your other leg over and rest your foot on your thigh. Lean forward, keep your back straight and reach for your toes.

Muscles being stretched
Primary muscles: Semimembranosus. Semitendinosus. Biceps femoris. Secondary muscle: Soleus.

Sports that benefit from this stretch
Basketball. Netball. Cycling. Hiking. Backpacking. Mountaineering. Orienteering. Ice hockey. Field hockey. Ice-skating. Roller-skating. Inline skating. Martial arts. Running. Track. Cross-country. American football (gridiron). Soccer. Rugby. Snow skiing. Water skiing. Surfing. Walking. Race walking. Wrestling.

Sports injury where stretch may be useful
Lower back muscle strain. Lower back ligament sprain. Hamstring strain. Calf strain.

Additional information for performing this stretch correctly
It is not important to be able to touch your toes. Simply reaching towards your toes is sufficient.

Complementary stretch
G07.

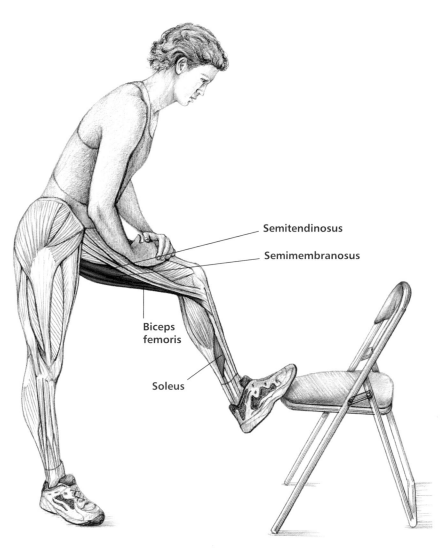

Semitendinosus

Semimembranosus

Biceps femoris

Soleus

Technique
Stand with one foot raised onto a chair or an object. Keep your leg slightly bent and let your heel drop off the edge of the object. Keep your back straight and move your chest towards your thigh.

Muscles being stretched
Primary muscles: Semimembranosus. Semitendinosus. Biceps femoris. Secondary muscle: Soleus.

Sports that benefit from this stretch
Basketball. Netball. Cycling. Hiking. Backpacking. Mountaineering. Orienteering. Ice hockey. Field hockey. Ice-skating. Roller-skating. Inline skating. Martial arts. Running. Track. Cross-country. American football (gridiron). Soccer. Rugby. Snow skiing. Water skiing. Surfing. Walking. Race walking. Wrestling.

Sports injury where stretch may be useful
Hamstring strain. Achilles tendon strain. Achilles tendonitis. Medial tibial pain syndrome (shin splints).

Additional information for performing this stretch correctly
Pushing your heel down towards the ground will help to intensify this stretch.

Complementary stretch
G14.

G13: STANDING HIGH-LEG BENT KNEE HAMSTRING STRETCH

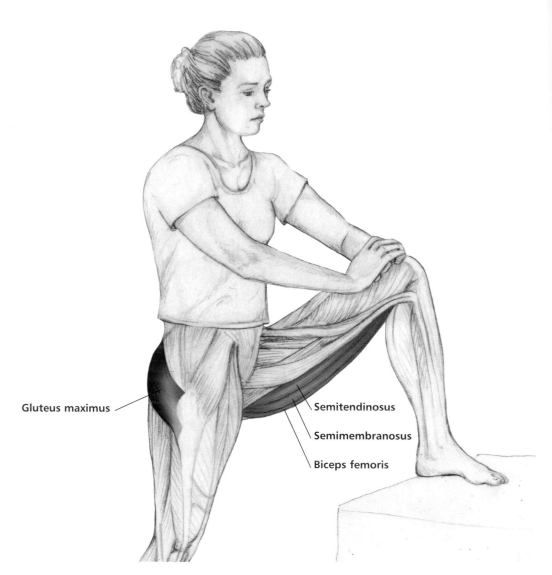

Gluteus maximus

Semitendinosus

Semimembranosus

Biceps femoris

Technique
Stand with one foot raised onto a table. Keep your leg bent and lean your chest into your bent knee.

Muscles being stretched
Primary muscle: Gluteus maximus.
Secondary muscles: Semimembranosus.
Semitendinosus. Biceps femoris.

Sports that benefit from this stretch
Basketball. Netball. Cycling. Hiking. Backpacking. Mountaineering. Orienteering. Ice hockey. Field hockey. Ice-skating. Roller-skating. Inline skating. Martial arts. Running. Track. Cross-country. Soccer. American football (gridiron). Rugby. Snow skiing. Water skiing. Surfing. Walking. Race walking. Wrestling.

Sports injury where stretch may be useful
Lower back muscle strain. Lower back ligament sprain. Hamstring strain.

Additional information for performing this stretch correctly
Regulate the intensity of this stretch by keeping your back straight and leaning forward.

Complementary stretches
G04, D08.

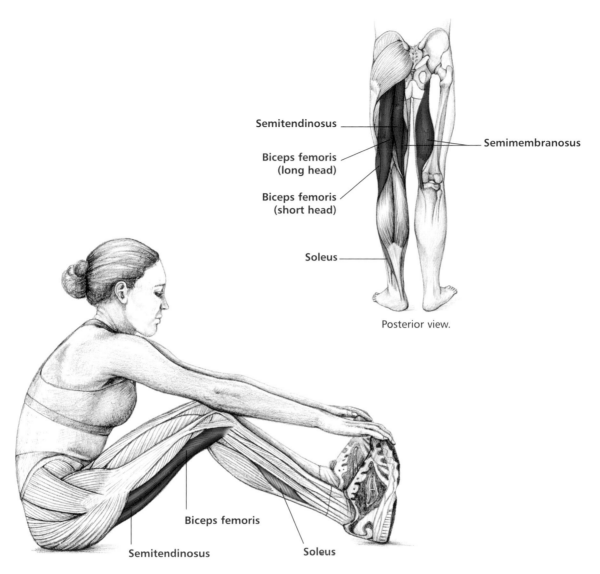

Semitendinosus

Semimembranosus

Biceps femoris
(long head)

Biceps femoris
(short head)

Soleus

Posterior view.

Biceps femoris

Semitendinosus

Soleus

Technique
Sit on the ground with your legs slightly bent.
Hold onto your toes with your hands and pull
your toes towards your body. Lean forward and
keep your back straight.

Muscles being stretched
Primary muscles: Semimembranosus.
Semitendinosus. Biceps femoris.
Secondary muscle: Soleus.

Sports that benefit from this stretch
Basketball. Netball. Cycling. Hiking. Backpacking.
Mountaineering. Orienteering. Ice hockey. Field
hockey. Ice-skating. Roller-skating. Inline skating.
Martial arts. Running. Track. Cross-country.
American football (gridiron). Soccer. Rugby. Snow
skiing. Water skiing. Surfing. Walking. Race
walking. Wrestling.

Sports injury where stretch may be useful
Hamstring strain. Achilles tendon strain.
Achilles tendonitis. Medial tibial pain
syndrome (shin splints).

Common problems and additional information for performing this stretch correctly
When pulling back on your toes, make sure
they are pointing straight upwards. Letting
your toes fall to one side will cause this stretch
to put uneven tension on the hamstring
muscles. Over an extended period of time, this
could lead to a muscle imbalance.

Complementary stretch
G08.

G15: STANDING REACH DOWN HAMSTRING STRETCH

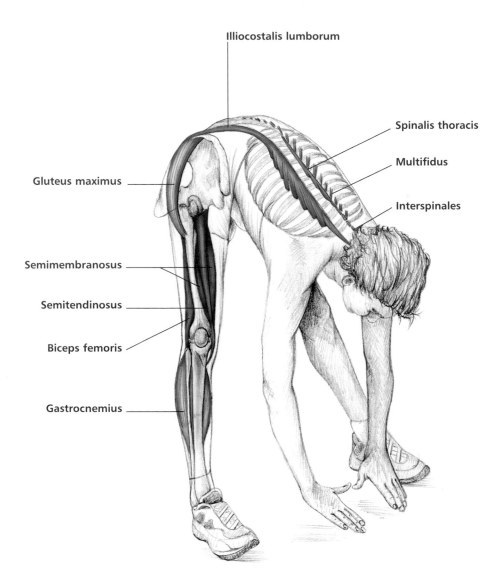

Illiocostalis lumborum

Spinalis thoracis

Multifidus

Interspinales

Gluteus maximus

Semimembranosus

Semitendinosus

Biceps femoris

Gastrocnemius

Technique
Stand with your feet shoulder-width apart. Bend forward and reach towards the ground.

Muscles being stretched
Primary muscles: Semimembranosus. Semitendinosus. Biceps femoris.
Secondary muscles: Gastrocnemius. Gluteus maximus. Iliocostalis lumborum. Spinalis thoracis. Interspinales. Multifidus.

Sports that benefit from this stretch
Basketball. Netball. Cycling. Hiking. Backpacking. Mountaineering. Orienteering. Ice hockey. Field hockey. Ice-skating. Roller-skating. Inline skating. Martial arts. Running. Track. Cross-country. American football (gridiron). Soccer. Rugby. Snow skiing. Water skiing. Surfing. Walking. Race walking. Wrestling.

Sports injury where stretch may be useful
Lower back muscle strain. Lower back ligament sprain. Hamstring strain. Calf strain.

Common problems and additional information for performing this stretch correctly
This position puts a lot of stress on the lower back muscles and the knees. Avoid this stretch if you have lower back pain or knee pain.

Complementary stretch
G01.

The adductors are a large group of muscles located on the medial (inner) side of the thigh. They originate at the bottom of the hip bone and extend down the inside of the thigh attaching to the medial side of the femur.

Pectineus is the most superior adductor; its primary action is adduction, or bringing the thigh toward the midline of the body. **Gracilis** attaches from the pubis symphysis to the tibia below the knee. It shapes the superficial inner thigh, but is relatively weak. It works the knee as well as the hip.

The three muscles specifically named adductors are the **adductor magnus**, **adductor brevis**, and **adductor longus**. They travel down the inside of the thigh, starting at the anterior pubis area of the pelvis and attaching to the medial length of the femur. The magnus is the largest of the three, and spreads out to cover the fullest area of the inside thigh.

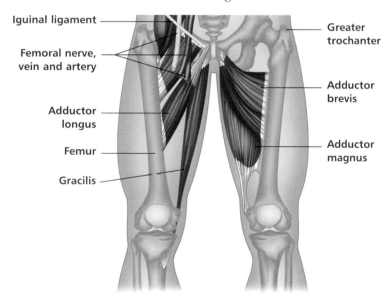

The primary action of the adductors is to adduct (draw towards the midline) the hip joint, but most also rotate the hip. The pectineus and gracilis inwardly rotate, and the adductor brevis and magnus outwardly rotate. All adductors function as stabilisers of the leg when weight is on it, and stabilise the pelvis.

Sports that benefit from these adductor stretches include: basketball and netball; cycling; hiking, backpacking, mountaineering, and orienteering; ice hockey and field hockey; ice-skating, roller-skating, and inline skating; martial arts; running, track, and cross-country; running sports like soccer, American football (gridiron), and rugby; snow skiing and water skiing; surfing; walking and race walking; wrestling.

H01: SITTING FEET TOGETHER ADDUCTOR STRETCH

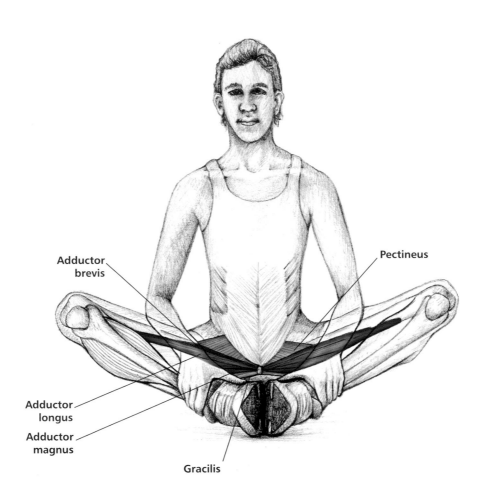

Adductor
brevis

Pectineus

Adductor
longus

Adductor
magnus

Gracilis

Technique
Sit with the soles of your feet together and bring your feet towards your groin. Hold onto your ankles and push your knee towards the ground with your elbows. Keep your back straight and upright.

Muscles being stretched
Primary muscles: Adductor longus, brevis, and magnus.
Secondary muscles: Gracilis. Pectineus.

Sports that benefit from this stretch
Basketball. Netball. Cycling. Hiking. Backpacking. Mountaineering. Orienteering. Ice hockey. Field hockey. Ice-skating. Roller-skating. Inline skating. Martial arts. Running. Track. Cross-country. American football (gridiron). Soccer. Rugby. Snow skiing. Water skiing. Surfing. Walking. Race walking. Wrestling.

Sports injury where stretch may be useful
Avulsion fracture in the pelvic area. Groin strain. Osteitis pubis. Piriformis syndrome. Tendonitis of the adductor muscles. Trochanteric bursitis.

Additional information for performing this stretch correctly
Keep your back straight and use your elbows to regulate the intensity of this stretch.

Complementary stretch
E08.

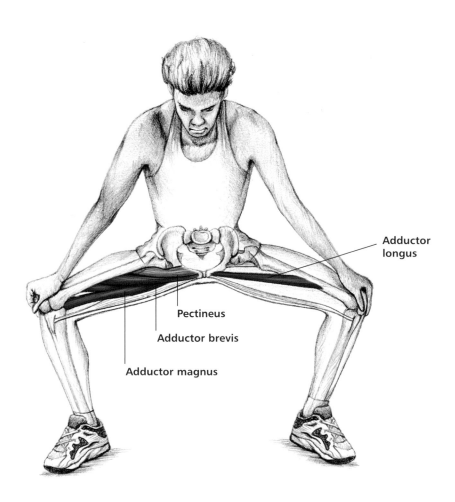

Adductor
longus

Pectineus

Adductor brevis

Adductor magnus

Technique
Stand with your feet wide apart and your toes pointing diagonally outwards. Bend at the knees, lean forward and use your hands to push your knees outwards.

Muscles being stretched
Primary muscles: Adductor longus, brevis, and magnus.
Secondary muscle: Pectineus.

Sports that benefit from this stretch
Basketball. Netball. Cycling. Hiking. Backpacking. Mountaineering. Orienteering. Ice hockey. Field hockey. Ice-skating. Roller-skating. Inline skating. Martial arts. Running. Track. Cross-country. American football (gridiron). Soccer. Rugby. Snow skiing. Water skiing. Surfing. Walking. Race walking. Wrestling.

Sports injury where stretch may be useful
Avulsion fracture in the pelvic area. Groin strain. Osteitis pubis. Piriformis syndrome. Tendonitis of the adductor muscles. Trochanteric bursitis.

Common problems and more information for performing this stretch correctly
Holding this position for extended periods of time requires a lot of quadriceps strength. If you start to feel your legs getting weak, take a break.

Complementary stretch
H07.

H03: STANDING LEG-UP ADDUCTOR STRETCH

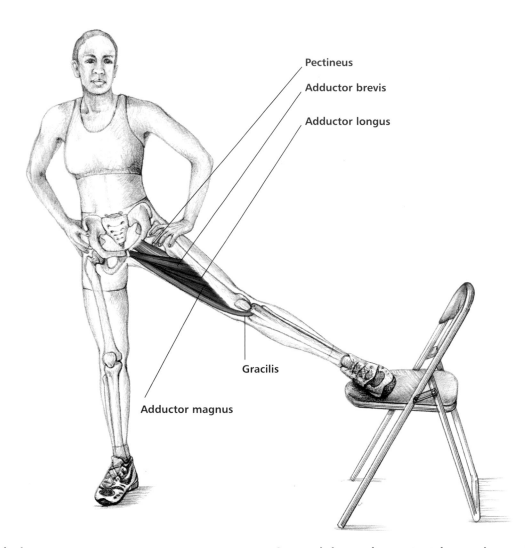

Pectineus

Adductor brevis

Adductor longus

Gracilis

Adductor magnus

Technique
Stand upright and place one leg out to the side and your foot up on a raised object. Keep your toes facing forward and slowly move your other leg away from the object.

Muscles being stretched
Primary muscles: Adductor longus, brevis, and magnus.
Secondary muscles: Gracilis. Pectineus.

Sports that benefit from this stretch
Basketball. Netball. Cycling. Hiking. Backpacking. Mountaineering. Orienteering. Ice hockey. Field hockey. Ice-skating. Roller-skating. Inline skating. Martial arts. Running. Track. Cross-country. American football (gridiron). Soccer. Rugby. Snow skiing. Water skiing. Surfing. Walking. Race walking. Wrestling.

Sports injury where stretch may be useful
Avulsion fracture in the pelvic area. Groin strain. Osteitis pubis. Piriformis syndrome. Tendonitis of the adductor muscles. Trochanteric bursitis.

Additional information for performing this stretch correctly
To increase the intensity of this stretch, use a higher object and if you need to, hold onto something for balance.

Complementary stretch
H01.

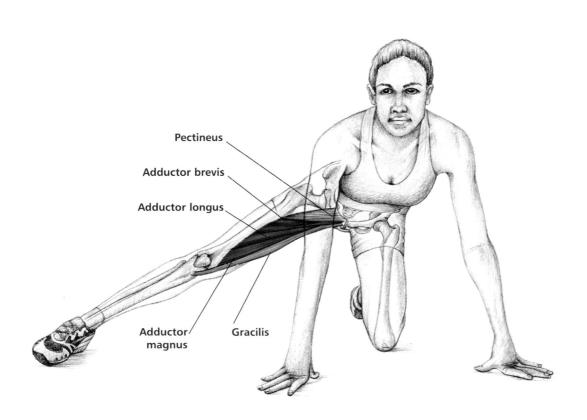

Pectineus

Adductor brevis

Adductor longus

Adductor magnus

Gracilis

Technique
Kneel on one knee and place your other leg out to the side with your toes facing forward. Rest your hands on the ground and slowly move your foot further out to the side.

Muscles being stretched
Primary muscles: Adductor longus, brevis, and magnus.
Secondary muscles: Gracilis. Pectineus.

Sports that benefit from this stretch
Basketball. Netball. Cycling. Hiking. Backpacking. Mountaineering. Orienteering. Ice hockey. Field hockey. Ice-skating. Roller-skating. Inline skating. Martial arts. Running. Track. Cross-country. American football (gridiron). Soccer. Rugby. Snow skiing. Water skiing. Surfing. Walking. Race walking. Wrestling.

Sports injury where stretch may be useful
Avulsion fracture in the pelvic area. Groin strain. Osteitis pubis. Piriformis syndrome. Tendonitis of the adductor muscles. Trochanteric bursitis.

Additional information for performing this stretch correctly
If need be, place a towel or mat under your knee for comfort.

Complementary stretch
H05.

H05: SQUATTING LEG-OUT ADDUCTOR STRETCH

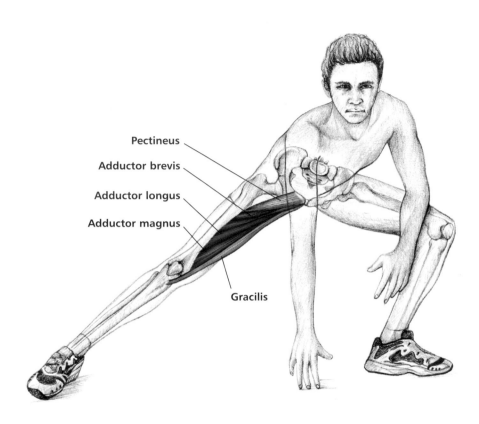

Pectineus

Adductor brevis

Adductor longus

Adductor magnus

Gracilis

Technique
Stand with your feet wide apart. Keep one leg straight and toes facing forward while bending the other leg and turning your toes out to the side. Lower your groin towards the ground and rest your hands on the bent knee or the ground.

Muscles being stretched
Primary muscles: Adductor longus, brevis, and magnus.
Secondary muscles: Gracilis. Pectineus.

Sports that benefit from this stretch
Basketball. Netball. Cycling. Hiking. Backpacking. Mountaineering. Orienteering. Ice hockey. Field hockey. Ice skating. Roller skating. Inline skating. Martial arts. Running. Track. Cross country. American football (gridiron). Soccer. Rugby. Snow skiing. Water skiing. Surfing. Walking. Race walking. Wrestling.

Sports injury where stretch may be useful
Avulsion fracture in the pelvic area. Groin strain. Osteitis pubis. Piriformis syndrome. Tendonitis of the adductor muscles. Trochanteric bursitis.

Additional information for performing this stretch correctly
Increase the intensity of this stretch by lowering yourself towards the ground.

Complementary stretch
H04.

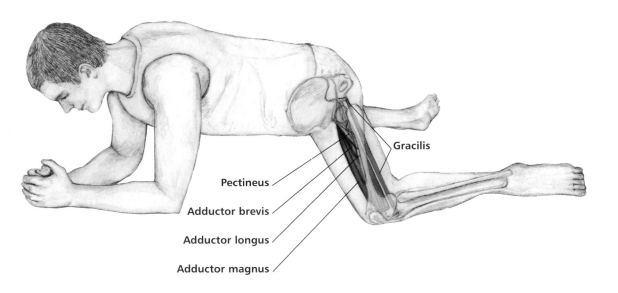

Gracilis

Pectineus

Adductor brevis

Adductor longus

Adductor magnus

Technique
Kneel face down with your knees and toes facing out. Lean forward and let your knees move outwards.

Muscles being stretched
Primary muscles: Adductor longus, brevis, and magnus.
Secondary muscles: Gracilis. Pectineus.

Sports that benefit from this stretch
Basketball. Netball. Cycling. Hiking. Backpacking. Mountaineering. Orienteering. Ice hockey. Field hockey. Ice-skating, Roller-skating. Inline skating. Martial arts. Running, Track. Cross-country. Soccer. American football (gridiron). Rugby. Snow skiing. Water skiing. Surfing. Walking. Race walking. Wrestling.

Sports injury where stretch may be useful
Avulsion fracture in the pelvic area. Groin strain. Osteitis pubis. Piriformis syndrome. Tendonitis of the adductor muscles. Trochanteric bursitis.

Additional information for performing this stretch correctly
Increase the intensity by lowering yourself towards the ground.

Complementary stretches
H01, H03.

H07: SITTING WIDE LEG ADDUCTOR STRETCH

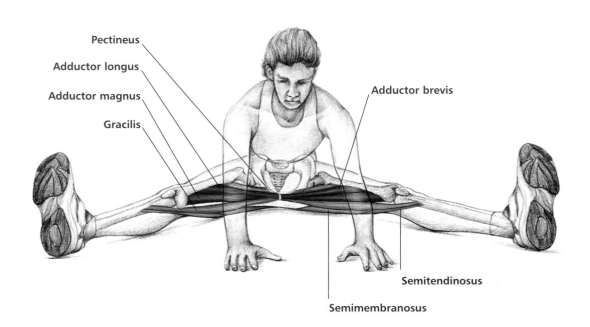

Pectineus

Adductor longus

Adductor magnus

Gracilis

Adductor brevis

Semitendinosus

Semimembranosus

Technique
Sit with your legs straight and wide apart. Keep your back straight and lean forward.

Muscles being stretched
Primary muscles: Adductor longus, brevis, and magnus.
Secondary muscles: Gracilis. Pectineus. Semimembranosus. Semitendinosus.

Sports that benefit from this stretch
Basketball. Netball. Cycling. Hiking. Backpacking. Mountaineering. Orienteering. Ice hockey. Field hockey. Ice-skating. Roller-skating. Inline skating. Martial arts. Running. Track. Cross-country. American football (gridiron). Soccer. Rugby. Snow skiing. Water skiing. Surfing. Walking. Race walking. Wrestling.

Sports injury where stretch may be useful
Avulsion fracture in the pelvic area. Groin strain. Osteitis pubis. Piriformis syndrome. Tendonitis of the adductor muscles. Trochanteric bursitis. Hamstring strain.

Additional information for performing this stretch correctly
To increase the intensity of this stretch, move your legs further apart.

Complementary stretch
H05.

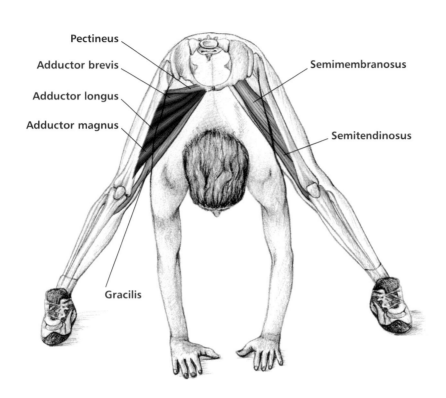

Pectineus

Adductor brevis

Adductor longus

Adductor magnus

Semimembranosus

Semitendinosus

Gracilis

Technique
Stand with your feet wide apart and your toes facing forward. Lean forward and reach towards the ground.

Muscles being stretched
Primary muscles: Adductor longus, brevis, and magnus.
Secondary muscles: Gracilis. Pectineus. Semimembranosus. Semitendinosus.

Sports that benefit from this stretch
Basketball. Netball. Cycling. Hiking. Backpacking. Mountaineering. Orienteering. Ice hockey. Field hockey. Ice-skating. Roller-skating. Inline skating. Martial arts. Running. Track. Cross-country. American football (gridiron). Soccer. Rugby. Snow skiing. Water skiing. Surfing. Walking. Race walking. Wrestling.

Sports injury where stretch may be useful
Avulsion fracture in the pelvic area. Groin strain. Osteitis pubis. Piriformis syndrome. Tendonitis of the adductor muscles. Trochanteric bursitis. Hamstring strain.

Common problems and more information for performing this stretch correctly
This position puts a lot of stress on the lower back muscles and the knees. Avoid this stretch if you have lower back pain or knee pain.

Complementary stretch
H03.

Abductors

The abductors are located on the lateral side (outside) of the thigh and hip. They originate at the top outer edge of the hip bone and extend down the outside of the thigh attaching to the lateral side of the tibia. The primary action of the abductors is to abduct (draw away from the midline) and medially rotate the hip joint.

Gluteus medius is mostly deep to and therefore obscured by gluteus maximus, but appears on the surface between gluteus maximus and tensor fasciae latae. During walking, gluteus medius, along with gluteus minimus, prevents the pelvis from dropping towards the non-weight bearing leg. When gluteus medius is tight, pelvic imbalances may result, leading to pain in the hips, lower back, and knees. **Gluteus minimus** lies deep to gluteus medius, whose fibers obscure it; as its name implies, it is the smallest of the gluteal muscles. As with gluteus medius, when minimus is tight, pelvic imbalances may occur.

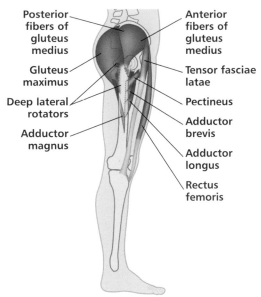

Posterior fibers of gluteus medius

Anterior fibers of gluteus medius

Gluteus maximus

Tensor fasciae latae

Deep lateral rotators

Pectineus

Adductor magnus

Adductor brevis

Adductor longus

Rectus femoris

Tensor fasciae latae lies anterior to gluteus maximus, and is a superficial muscle of the upper thigh that keeps your pelvis level, and stabilises your knee as you stand on one leg. It also assists in flexion of the hip joint.

Sports that benefit from these abductor stretches include: cycling; hiking, backpacking, mountaineering, and orienteering; ice hockey and field hockey; ice-skating, roller-skating, and inline skating; martial arts; rowing, canoeing, and kayaking; running, track, and cross-country; running sports like soccer, American football (gridiron), and rugby; snow skiing and water skiing; walking and race walking.

I01: STANDING HIP-OUT ABDUCTOR STRETCH

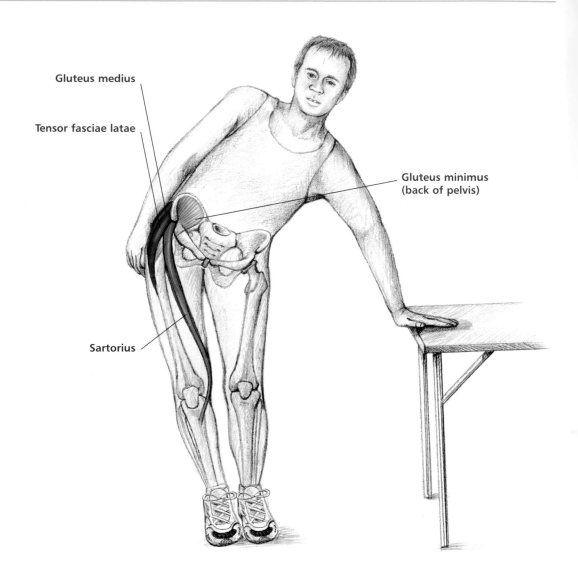

Gluteus medius

Tensor fasciae latae

Gluteus minimus
(back of pelvis)

Sartorius

Technique
Stand upright beside a wall or table with both feet together. Lean your upper body towards the wall and push your hips away from the wall. Keep your outside leg straight and your inside leg slightly bent.

Muscles being stretched
Primary muscles: Tensor fasciae latae. Gluteus medius and minimus.
Secondary muscle: Sartorius.

Sports that benefit from this stretch
Basketball. Netball. Cycling. Hiking. Backpacking. Mountaineering. Orienteering. Ice hockey. Field hockey. Ice-skating. Roller-skating. Inline skating. Martial arts. Running. Track. Cross-country. American football (gridiron). Soccer. Rugby. Snow skiing. Water skiing. Surfing. Walking. Race walking. Wrestling.

Sports injury where stretch may be useful
Trochanteric bursitis. Iliotibial band syndrome.

Common problems and more information for performing this stretch correctly
It is important not to bend forward during this stretch. Keep your body upright and concentrate on pushing your hips away from the object you're leaning on.

Complementary stretch
I07.

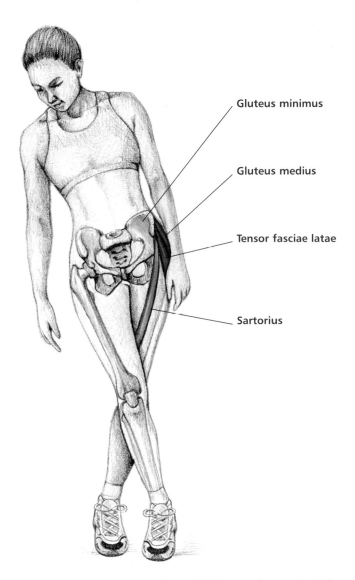

Gluteus minimus

Gluteus medius

Tensor fasciae latae

Sartorius

Technique
Stand upright and cross one foot behind the other. Lean towards the foot that is behind the other.

Muscles being stretched
Primary muscles: Tensor fasciae latae. Gluteus medius and minimus.
Secondary muscle: Sartorius.

Sports that benefit from this stretch
Basketball. Netball. Cycling. Hiking. Backpacking. Mountaineering. Orienteering. Ice hockey. Field hockey. Ice-skating. Roller-skating. Inline skating. Martial arts. Running. Track. Cross-country. American football (gridiron). Soccer. Rugby. Snow skiing. Water skiing. Surfing. Walking. Race walking. Wrestling.

Sports injury where stretch may be useful
Trochanteric bursitis. Iliotibial band syndrome.

Additional information for performing this stretch correctly
If need be, hold onto something for balance. This will allow you to concentrate on the stretch, instead of worrying about falling over.

Complementary stretch
D21.

103: LEANING ABDUCTOR STRETCH

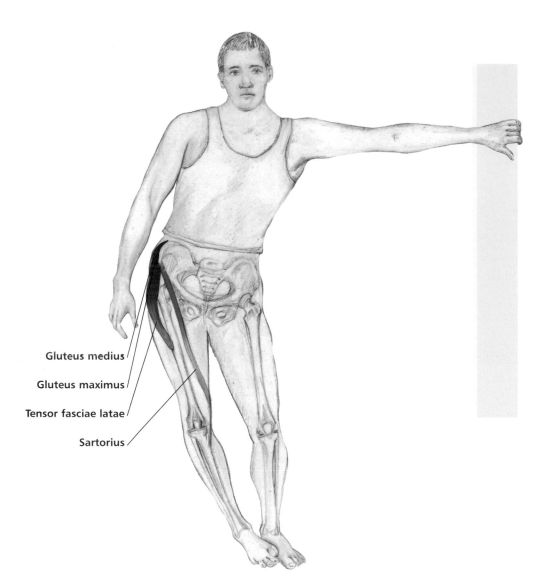

Gluteus medius

Gluteus maximus

Tensor fasciae latae

Sartorius

Technique
Hold onto the pole with one hand, while standing next to a pole or door jam. Keep your feet together, and lean your hips away from the pole. Keep your outside leg straight and bend your inside leg slightly.

Muscles being stretched
Primary muscles: Tensor fasciae latae. Gluteus medius and mininus.
Secondary muscle: Sartorius.

Sports that benefit from this stretch
Basketball. Netball. Cycling. Hiking. Backpacking. Mountaineering. Orienteering. Ice hockey. Field hockey. Ice-skating. Roller-skating. Inline skating. Martial arts. Running. Track. Cross-country. Soccer. American football (gridiron). Rugby. Snow skiing. Water skiing. Surfing. Walking. Race walking. Wrestling.

Sports injury where stretch may be useful
Trochanteric bursitis. Iliotibial band syndrome.

Common problems and more information for performing this stretch correctly
It is important not to bend forward during this stretch. Keep your body upright and concentrate on pushing your hips away from the object you are holding on to.

Complementary stretch
104.

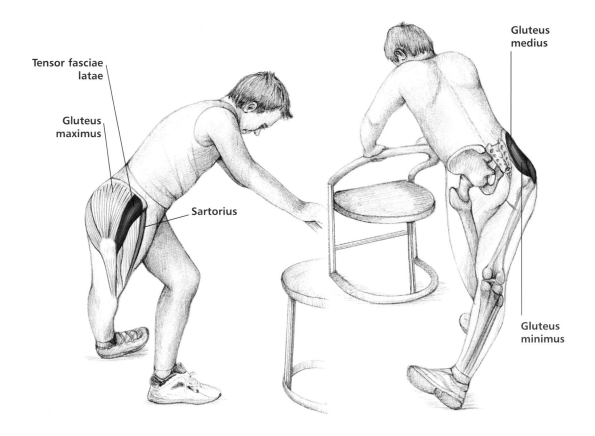

Tensor fasciae latae

Gluteus maximus

Sartorius

Gluteus medius

Gluteus minimus

Technique
While standing, lean forward and hold onto a chair or bench to help with balance. Cross one foot behind the other and slide that foot away from your body, keeping your leg straight. Slowly bend your front leg to lower your body.

Muscles being stretched
Primary muscles: Tensor fasciae latae. Gluteus medius and mininus.
Secondary muscle: Sartorius.

Sports that benefit from this stretch
Basketball. Netball. Cycling. Hiking. Backpacking. Mountaineering. Orienteering. Ice hockey. Field hockey. Ice-skating. Roller-skating. Inline skating. Martial arts. Running. Track. Cross-country. American football (gridiron). Soccer. Rugby. Snow skiing. Water skiing. Surfing. Walking. Race walking. Wrestling.

Sports injury where stretch may be useful
Trochanteric bursitis. Iliotibial band syndrome.

Additional information for performing this stretch correctly
Regulate the intensity of the stretch by using your bent leg to lower your body.

Complementary stretch
102.

I05: LYING ABDUCTOR STRETCH

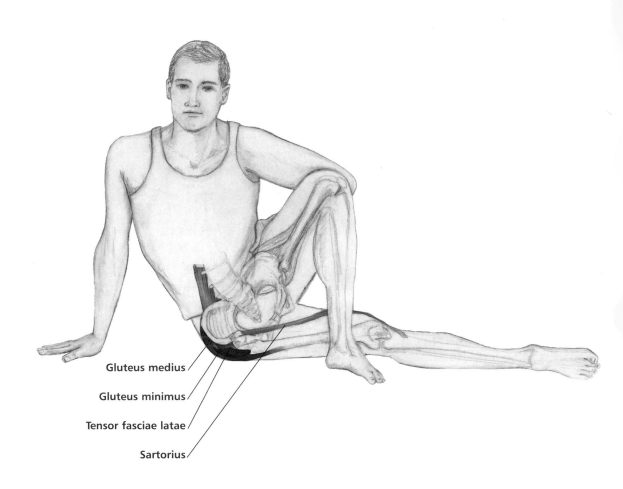

Gluteus medius

Gluteus minimus

Tensor fasciae latae

Sartorius

Technique
Lean on your side on the ground and bring your top leg up to your other knee. Push your body up with your arm and keep your hip on the ground.

Muscles being stretched
Primary muscles: Tensor fasciae latae. Gluteus medius and mininus.
Secondary muscles: Sartorius. Quadratus lumborum.

Sports that benefit from this stretch
Basketball. Netball. Cycling. Hiking. Backpacking. Mountaineering. Orienteering. Ice hockey. Field hockey. Ice-skating. Roller-skating. Inline skating. Martial arts. Running. Track. Cross-country. Soccer. American football (gridiron). Rugby. Snow skiing. Water skiing. Surfing. Walking. Race walking. Wrestling.

Sports injury where stretch may be useful
Trochanteric bursitis. Iliotibial band syndrome.

Common problems and more information for performing this stretch correctly
Increase the intensity of this stretch by lowering yourself towards the ground.

Complementary stretches
I02, I04.

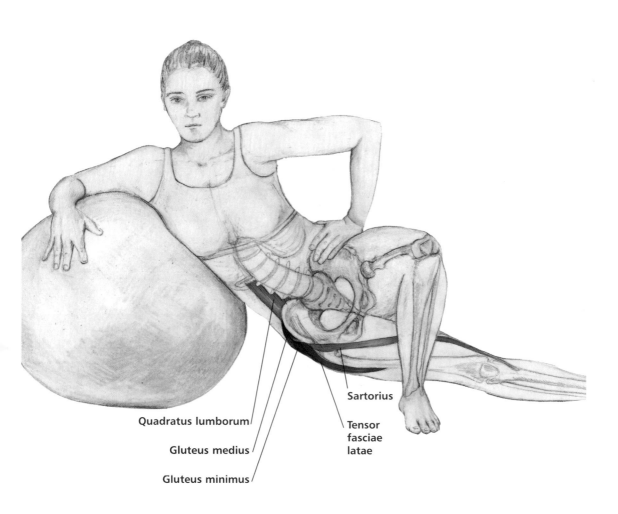

Quadratus lumborum

Gluteus medius

Gluteus minimus

Sartorius

Tensor fasciae latae

Technique
Lean on your side on a Swiss ball and place one leg straight out to the side. Bring your top leg up to your other knee and push your hip towards the ground.

Muscles being stretched
Primary muscles: Tensor fasciae latae. Gluteus medius and mininus.
Secondary muscles: Sartorius. Quadratus lumborum.

Sports that benefit from this stretch
Basketball. Netball. Cycling. Hiking. Backpacking. Mountaineering. Orienteering. Ice hockey. Field hockey. Ice-skating. Roller-skating. Inline skating. Martial arts. Running. Track. Cross-country. Soccer. American football (gridiron). Rugby. Snow skiing. Water skiing. Surfing. Walking. Race walking. Wrestling.

Sports injury where stretch may be useful
Trochanteric bursitis. Iliotibial band syndrome.

Common problems and more information for performing this stretch correctly
It is important not to bend forward during this stretch. Keep your body upright and regulate the intensity of the stretch by pushing your hips down and your torso into a more upright position.

Complementary stretches
103, 107.

107: LYING LEG HANG ABDUCTOR STRETCH

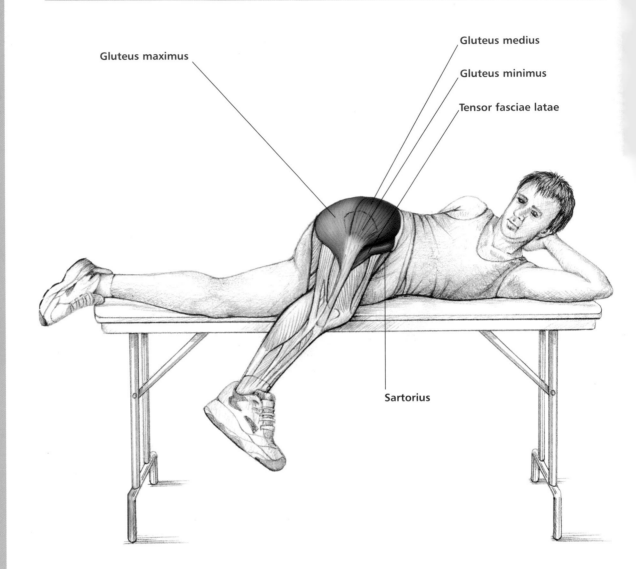

Gluteus maximus

Gluteus medius

Gluteus minimus

Tensor fasciae latae

Sartorius

Technique
Lie on a bench on your side. Allow the top leg to fall forward and off the side of the bench.

Muscles being stretched
Primary muscles: Tensor fasciae latae. Gluteus medius and mininus.
Secondary muscles: Sartorius. Gluteus maximus.

Sports that benefit from this stretch
Basketball. Netball. Cycling. Hiking. Backpacking. Mountaineering. Orienteering. Ice hockey. Field hockey. Ice-skating. Roller-skating. Inline skating. Martial arts. Running. Track. Cross-country. American football (gridiron). Soccer. Rugby. Snow skiing. Water skiing. Surfing. Walking. Race walking. Wrestling.

Sports injury where stretch may be useful
Trochanteric bursitis. Iliotibial band syndrome.

Common problems and more information for performing this stretch correctly
Try not to let your leg fall too far forward and use the weight of your leg to do the stretching for you.

Complementary stretch
E09.

12 Upper Calves

The upper calf muscles are located on the posterior (rear) of the lower leg just underneath the knee joint. They originate at the bottom of the femur, just above the knee joint, and extend down into the Achilles tendon. The primary actions of the upper calf muscles are to plantar flex the ankle joint and flex the knee.

Plantaris is a small muscle, which is a weak plantar flexor of the ankle, but plays an important neurological role in assessing and adjusting the tension in the Achilles tendon. The long slender tendon of plantaris is equivalent to the tendon of palmaris longus in the arm. Interestingly, plantaris is thought to be what remains of a larger plantar flexor of the foot.

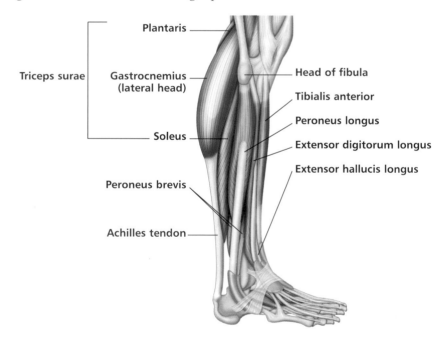

The superficial **gastrocnemius** has two heads and crosses two joints: the knee and the ankle. It is part of the composite muscle known as *triceps surae*, which forms the prominent contour of the calf. The triceps surae comprises: gastrocnemius, soleus, and plantaris. Gastrocnemius is quite a thin muscle when compared to the thick soleus. (Soleus is featured in Chapter 13.) As well as plantar flexing the ankle, gastrocnemius assists in flexion of the knee joint, and is a main propelling force in walking and running. Explosive sprinting, for example, may rupture the Achilles tendon at its junction with the muscle belly of gastrocnemius, hence the need to keep it well stretched.

Sports that benefit from these upper calf stretches include: basketball and netball; boxing; cycling; hiking, backpacking, mountaineering, and orienteering; ice hockey and field hockey; ice-skating, roller-skating, and inline skating; martial arts; racquet sports like tennis, badminton, and squash; running, track, and cross-country; running sports like soccer, American football (gridiron), and rugby; snow skiing and water skiing; surfing; swimming; walking and race walking.

J01: STANDING TOE-UP CALF STRETCH

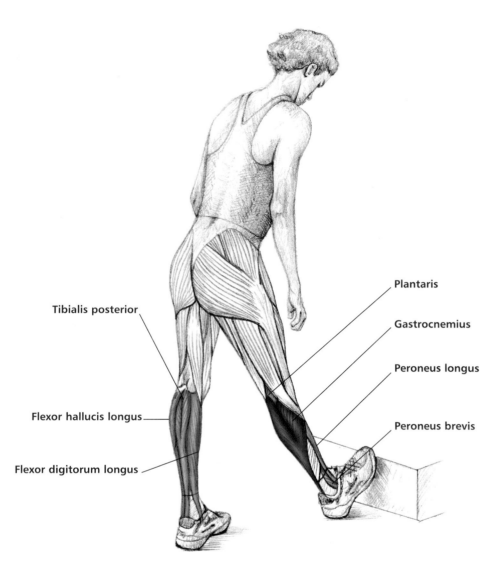

Tibialis posterior

Flexor hallucis longus

Flexor digitorum longus

Plantaris

Gastrocnemius

Peroneus longus

Peroneus brevis

Technique
Stand upright and place your toes on a step or raised object. Keep your leg straight and lean towards your toes.

Muscles being stretched
Primary muscle: Gastrocnemius.
Secondary muscles: Tibialis posterior. Flexor hallucis longus. Flexor digitorum longus. Peroneus longus and brevis. Plantaris.

Sports that benefit from this stretch
Basketball. Netball. Boxing. Cycling. Hiking. Backpacking. Mountaineering. Orienteering. Ice hockey. Field hockey. Ice-skating. Roller-skating. Inline skating. Martial arts. Tennis. Badminton. Squash. Running. Track. Cross-country. American football (gridiron). Soccer. Rugby. Snow skiing. Water skiing. Surfing. Swimming. Walking. Race walking.

Sports injury where stretch may be useful
Calf strain. Achilles tendon strain. Achilles tendonitis. Medial tibial pain syndrome (shin splints).

Additional information for performing this stretch correctly
Regulate the intensity of this stretch by keeping your back straight and leaning forward.

Complementary stretch
J03.

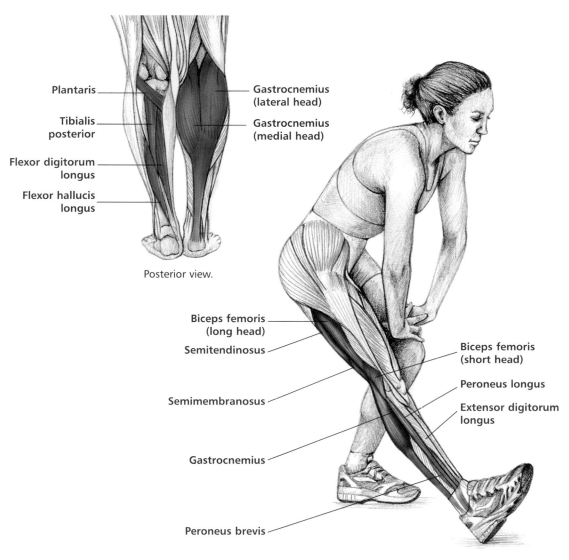

Plantaris

Tibialis posterior

Flexor digitorum longus

Flexor hallucis longus

Gastrocnemius (lateral head)

Gastrocnemius (medial head)

Posterior view.

Biceps femoris (long head)

Semitendinosus

Semimembranosus

Gastrocnemius

Peroneus brevis

Biceps femoris (short head)

Peroneus longus

Extensor digitorum longus

Technique
Stand with one knee bent and the other leg straight out in front. Point your toes towards your body and lean forward. Keep your back straight and rest your hands on your bent knee.

Muscles being stretched
Primary muscles: Gastrocnemius. Semimembranosus. Semitendinosus. Biceps femoris.
Secondary muscles: Tibialis posterior. Flexor hallucis longus. Flexor digitorum longus. Peroneus longus and brevis. Plantaris.

Sports that benefit from this stretch
Basketball. Netball. Boxing. Cycling. Hiking. Backpacking. Mountaineering. Orienteering. Ice hockey. Field hockey. Ice-skating. Roller-skating. Inline skating. Martial arts. Tennis. Badminton. Squash. Running. Track. Cross-country. American football (gridiron). Soccer. Rugby. Snow skiing. Water skiing. Surfing. Swimming. Walking. Race walking.

Sports injury where stretch may be useful
Hamstring strain. Calf strain. Achilles tendon strain. Achilles tendonitis. Medial tibial pain syndrome (shin splints).

Common problems and more information for performing this stretch correctly
Make sure your toes are pointing upward. Letting your toes point to one side will cause this stretch to put uneven tension on the calf muscles. Over an extended period of time, this could lead to a muscle imbalance.

Complementary stretch
J04.

J03: SINGLE HEEL DROP CALF STRETCH

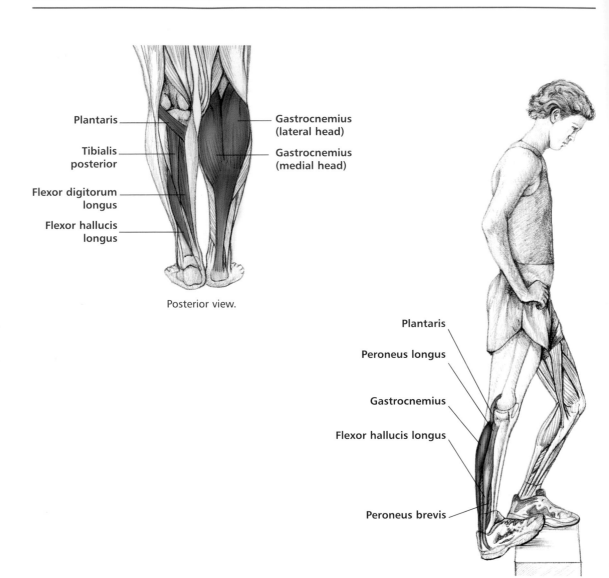

Plantaris

Tibialis posterior

Flexor digitorum longus

Flexor hallucis longus

Gastrocnemius (lateral head)

Gastrocnemius (medial head)

Posterior view.

Plantaris

Peroneus longus

Gastrocnemius

Flexor hallucis longus

Peroneus brevis

Technique
Stand on a raised object or step. Put the toes of one foot on the edge of the step and keep your leg straight. Let your heel drop towards the ground.

Muscles being stretched
Primary muscle: Gastrocnemius.
Secondary muscles: Tibialis posterior. Flexor hallucis longus. Flexor digitorum longus. Peroneus longus and brevis. Plantaris.

Sports that benefit from this stretch
Basketball. Netball. Boxing. Cycling. Hiking. Backpacking. Mountaineering. Orienteering. Ice hockey. Field hockey. Ice-skating. Roller-skating. Inline skating. Martial arts. Tennis. Badminton. Squash. Running. Track. Cross-country. American football (gridiron). Soccer. Rugby. Snow skiing. Water skiing. Surfing. Swimming. Walking. Race walking.

Sports injury where stretch may be useful
Calf strain. Achilles tendon strain. Achilles tendonitis. Medial tibial pain syndrome (shin splints).

Common problems and more information for performing this stretch correctly
This stretch can put a lot of pressure on the Achilles tendon. Ease into this stretch by slowly lowering your heel.

Complementary stretch
J02.

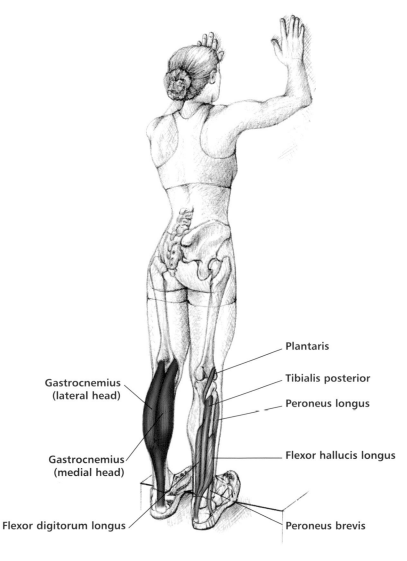

Plantaris

Tibialis posterior

Peroneus longus

Flexor hallucis longus

Gastrocnemius
(lateral head)

Gastrocnemius
(medial head)

Flexor digitorum longus

Peroneus brevis

Technique
Stand on a raised object or step. Put the toes of both of your feet on the edge of the step and keep your legs straight. Let your heels drop towards the ground and lean forward.

Muscles being stretched
Primary muscle: Gastrocnemius. Secondary muscles: Tibialis posterior. Flexor hallucis longus. Flexor digitorum longus. Peroneus longus and brevis. Plantaris.

Sports that benefit from this stretch
Basketball. Netball. Boxing. Cycling. Hiking. Backpacking. Mountaineering. Orienteering. Ice hockey. Field hockey. Ice-skating. Roller-skating. Inline skating. Martial arts. Tennis. Badminton. Squash. Running. Track. Cross-country. American football (gridiron). Soccer. Rugby. Snow skiing. Water skiing. Surfing. Swimming. Walking. Race walking.

Sports injury where stretch may be useful
Calf strain. Achilles tendon strain. Achilles tendonitis. Medial tibial pain syndrome (shin splints).

Additional information for performing this stretch correctly
Let your body weight regulate the intensity of this stretch.

Complementary stretch
J06.

J05: STANDING HEEL BACK CALF STRETCH

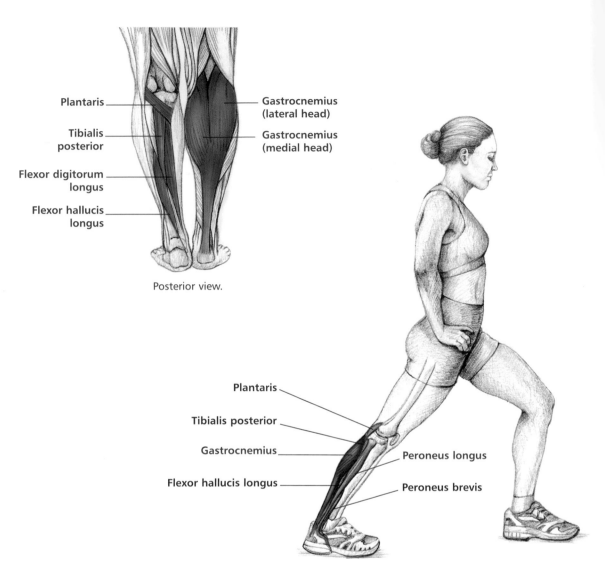

Plantaris

Gastrocnemius (lateral head)

Tibialis posterior

Gastrocnemius (medial head)

Flexor digitorum longus

Flexor hallucis longus

Posterior view.

Plantaris

Tibialis posterior

Gastrocnemius

Peroneus longus

Flexor hallucis longus

Peroneus brevis

Technique
Stand upright and then take one big step backwards. Keep your back leg straight and push your heel to the ground.

Muscles being stretched
Primary muscle: Gastrocnemius.
Secondary muscles: Tibialis posterior. Flexor hallucis longus. Flexor digitorum longus. Peroneus longus and brevis. Plantaris.

Sports that benefit from this stretch
Basketball. Netball. Boxing. Cycling. Hiking. Backpacking. Mountaineering. Orienteering. Ice hockey. Field hockey. Ice-skating. Roller-skating. Inline skating. Martial arts. Tennis. Badminton. Squash. Running. Track. Cross-country. American football (gridiron). Soccer. Rugby. Snow skiing. Water skiing. Surfing. Swimming. Walking. Race walking.

Sports injury where stretch may be useful
Calf strain. Achilles tendon strain. Achilles tendonitis. Medial tibial pain syndrome (shin splints).

Common problems and more information for performing this stretch correctly
Make sure that the toes of your back leg are facing forward. Letting your toes point to one side will cause this stretch to put uneven tension on the calf muscles. Over an extended period of time, this could lead to a muscle imbalance.

Complementary stretch
J01.

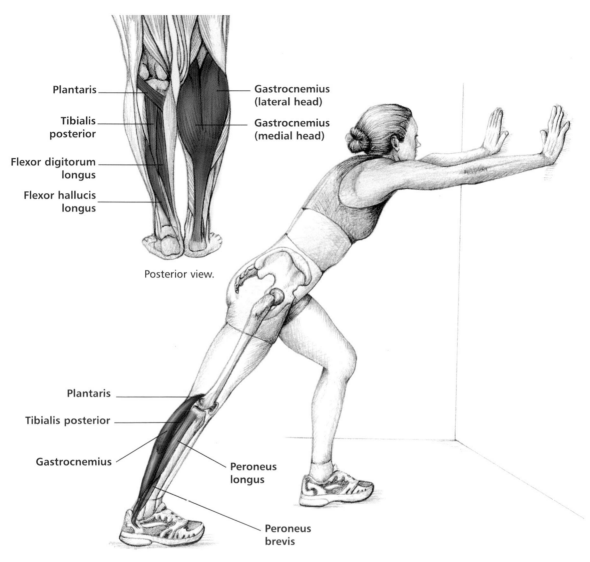

Plantaris

Tibialis posterior

Flexor digitorum longus

Flexor hallucis longus

Gastrocnemius (lateral head)

Gastrocnemius (medial head)

Posterior view.

Plantaris

Tibialis posterior

Gastrocnemius

Peroneus longus

Peroneus brevis

Technique
Stand upright and lean against a wall. Place one foot as far from the wall as is comfortable and make sure that both toes are facing forward and your heel is on the ground. Keep your back leg straight and lean towards the wall.

Muscles being stretched
Primary muscle: Gastrocnemius.
Secondary muscles: Tibialis posterior. Flexor hallucis longus. Flexor digitorum longus. Peroneus longus and brevis. Plantaris.

Sports that benefit from this stretch
Basketball. Netball. Boxing. Cycling. Hiking. Backpacking. Mountaineering. Orienteering. Ice hockey. Field hockey. Ice-skating. Roller-skating. Inline skating. Martial arts. Tennis. Badminton. Squash. Running. Track. Cross-country. American football (gridiron). Soccer. Rugby. Snow skiing. Water skiing. Surfing. Swimming. Walking. Race walking.

Sports injury where stretch may be useful
Calf strain. Achilles tendon strain. Achilles tendonitis. Medial tibial pain syndrome (shin splints).

Common problems and more information for performing this stretch correctly
Make sure the toes of your back leg are facing forward. Letting your toes point to one side will cause this stretch to put uneven tension on the calf muscles. Over an extended period of time, this could lead to a muscle imbalance.

Complementary stretch
J02.

J07: CROUCHING HEEL BACK CALF STRETCH

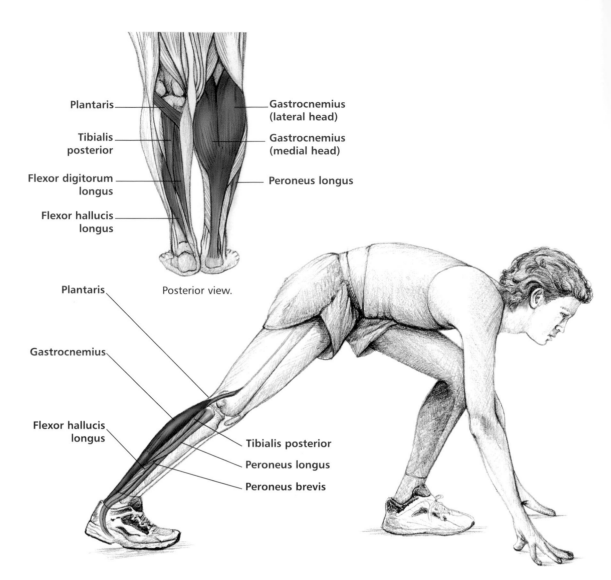

Plantaris

Tibialis posterior

Flexor digitorum longus

Flexor hallucis longus

Gastrocnemius (lateral head)

Gastrocnemius (medial head)

Peroneus longus

Posterior view.

Plantaris

Gastrocnemius

Flexor hallucis longus

Tibialis posterior

Peroneus longus

Peroneus brevis

Technique
Stand upright and place one foot in front of the other. Bend your front leg and keep your back leg straight. Push your heel to the ground and lean forward. Place your hands on the ground in front of you.

Muscles being stretched
Primary muscle: Gastrocnemius.
Secondary muscles: Tibialis posterior. Flexor hallucis longus. Flexor digitorum longus. Peroneus longus and brevis. Plantaris.

Sports that benefit from this stretch
Basketball. Netball. Boxing. Cycling. Hiking. Backpacking. Mountaineering. Orienteering. Ice hockey. Field hockey. Ice-skating. Roller-skating. Inline skating. Martial arts. Tennis. Badminton. Squash. Running. Track. Cross-country. American football (gridiron). Soccer. Rugby. Snow skiing. Water skiing. Surfing. Swimming. Walking. Race walking.

Sports injury where stretch may be useful
Calf strain. Achilles tendon strain. Achilles tendonitis. Medial tibial pain syndrome (shin splints).

Common problems and more information for performing this stretch correctly
Make sure the toes of your back leg are facing forward. Letting your toes point to one side will cause this stretch to put uneven tension on the calf muscles. Over an extended period of time, this could lead to a muscle imbalance.

Complementary stretch
J04.

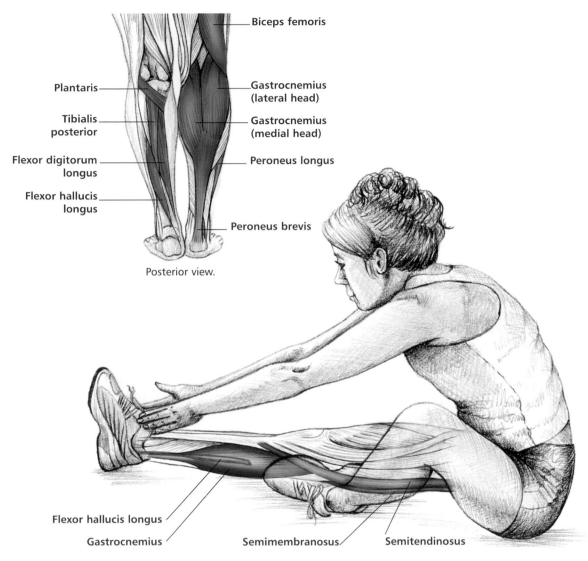

Biceps femoris

Plantaris

Gastrocnemius
(lateral head)

Tibialis
posterior

Gastrocnemius
(medial head)

Flexor digitorum
longus

Peroneus longus

Flexor hallucis
longus

Peroneus brevis

Posterior view.

Flexor hallucis longus

Gastrocnemius

Semimembranosus

Semitendinosus

Technique
Sit with one leg straight and your toes pointing up. Lean forward and pull your toes back towards your body.

Muscles being stretched
Primary muscles: Gastrocnemius. Semimembranosus. Semitendinosus. Biceps femoris.
Secondary muscles: Tibialis posterior. Flexor hallucis longus. Flexor digitorum longus. Peroneus longus and brevis. Plantaris.

Sports that benefit from this stretch
Basketball. Netball. Boxing. Cycling. Hiking. Backpacking. Mountaineering. Orienteering. Ice hockey. Field hockey. Ice-skating. Roller-skating. Inline skating. Martial arts. Tennis. Badminton. Squash. Running. Track. Cross-country. American football (gridiron). Soccer. Rugby. Snow skiing. Water skiing. Surfing. Swimming. Walking. Race walking.

Sports injury where stretch may be useful
Hamstring strain. Calf strain. Achilles tendon strain. Achilles tendonitis. Medial tibial pain syndrome (shin splints).

Common problems and more information for performing this stretch correctly
If you have trouble reaching your toes in this position, avoid this stretch.

Complementary stretch
J07.

Lower Calves and Achilles Tendon

The lower calf muscles are located on the posterior (rear) of the lower leg below the knee joint. They originate at the top of the tibia, just below the knee joint, and extend down into the Achilles tendon. The primary action of the lower calf muscles is to plantar flex the ankle joint.

Peroneus (fibularis) longus and **peroneus (fibularis) brevis** form the lateral compartment of the lower calf. Both these muscles act as plantar flexors and everters at the ankle joint, but also as preventers of inversion and protectors against ankle sprain. The course of the tendon of insertion of peroneus (fibularis) longus helps maintain the transverse and lateral longitudinal arches of the foot.

Flexor digitorum longus, **flexor hallucis longus**, and **tibialis posterior** form the deep posterior compartment of the lower leg. Tibialis posterior is the deepest muscle and helps maintain the arches of the foot. Flexor hallucis longus helps maintain the medial longitudinal arch of the foot.

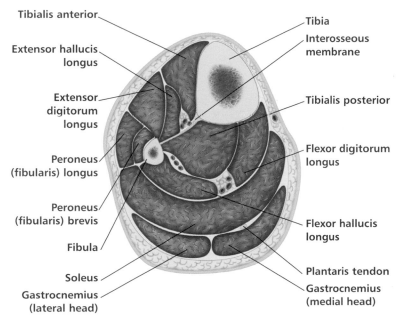

Tibialis anterior

Extensor hallucis longus

Extensor digitorum longus

Peroneus (fibularis) longus

Peroneus (fibularis) brevis

Fibula

Soleus

Gastrocnemius (lateral head)

Tibia

Interosseous membrane

Tibialis posterior

Flexor digitorum longus

Flexor hallucis longus

Plantaris tendon

Gastrocnemius (medial head)

Part of the triceps surae, **soleus** is so-called because its shape resembles a fish. It is deep to gastrocnemius, but its medial and lateral fibers bulge from the sides of the leg and extend further distal than gastrocnemius. Constant wearing of high-heeled shoes tends to cause this muscle to shorten, which can affect postural integrity.

Sports that benefit from these lower calf stretches include: basketball and netball; boxing; cycling; hiking, backpacking, mountaineering, and orienteering; ice hockey and field hockey; ice-skating, roller-skating, and inline skating; martial arts; racquet sports like tennis, badminton, and squash; running, track, and cross-country; running sports like soccer, American football (gridiron), and rugby; snow skiing and water skiing; surfing; swimming; walking and race walking.

K01: STANDING TOE-UP ACHILLES STRETCH

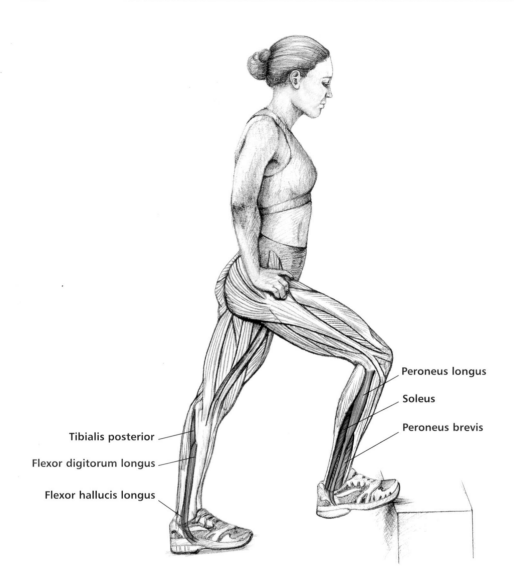

Peroneus longus

Soleus

Peroneus brevis

Tibialis posterior

Flexor digitorum longus

Flexor hallucis longus

Technique
Stand upright and place your toes against a step or raised object. Bend your leg and lean towards your toes.

Muscles being stretched
Primary muscle: Soleus.
Secondary muscles: Tibialis posterior. Flexor hallucis longus. Flexor digitorum longus. Peroneus longus and brevis.

Sports that benefit from this stretch
Basketball. Netball. Boxing. Cycling. Hiking. Backpacking. Mountaineering. Orienteering. Ice hockey. Field hockey. Ice-skating. Roller-skating. Inline skating. Martial arts. Tennis. Badminton. Squash. Running. Track. Cross-country. American football (gridiron). Soccer. Rugby. Snow skiing. Water skiing. Surfing. Swimming. Walking. Race walking.

Sports injury where stretch may be useful
Calf strain. Achilles tendon strain. Achilles tendonitis. Medial tibial pain syndrome (shin splints). Posterior tibial tendonitis.

Additional information for performing this stretch correctly
Regulate the intensity of this stretch by relaxing your calf muscles and pushing your heel to the ground.

Complementary stretch
K03.

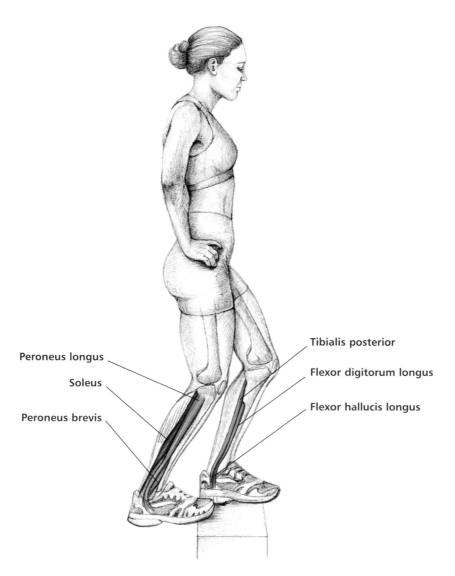

Peroneus longus

Soleus

Peroneus brevis

Tibialis posterior

Flexor digitorum longus

Flexor hallucis longus

Technique
Stand on a raised object or step and place the toes of one of your feet on the edge of the step. Bend your leg and let your heel drop towards the ground.

Muscles being stretched
Primary muscle: Soleus.
Secondary muscles: Tibialis posterior. Flexor hallucis longus. Flexor digitorum longus. Peroneus longus and brevis.

Sports that benefit from this stretch
Basketball. Netball. Boxing. Cycling. Hiking. Backpacking. Mountaineering. Orienteering. Ice hockey. Field hockey. Ice-skating. Roller-skating. Inline skating. Martial arts. Tennis. Badminton. Squash. Running. Track. Cross-country. American football (gridiron). Soccer. Rugby. Snow skiing. Water skiing. Surfing. Swimming. Walking. Race walking.

Sports injury where stretch may be useful
Calf strain. Achilles tendon strain. Achilles tendonitis. Medial tibial pain syndrome (shin splints). Posterior tibial tendonitis.

Common problems and more information for performing this stretch correctly
This stretch can put a lot of pressure on the Achilles tendon. Ease into this stretch by slowly lowering your heel.

Complementary stretch
K04.

K03: STANDING HEEL BACK ACHILLES STRETCH

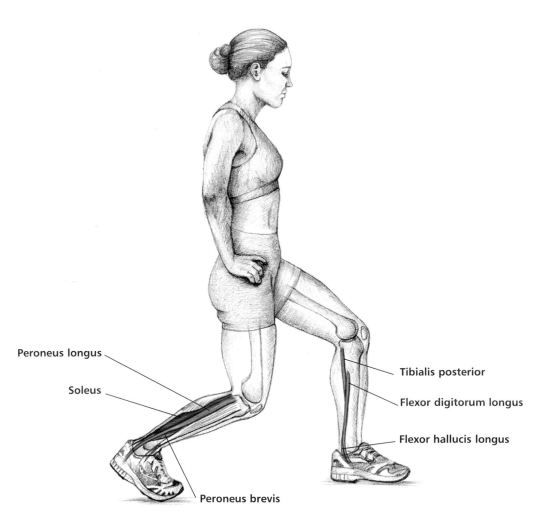

Peroneus longus

Soleus

Tibialis posterior

Flexor digitorum longus

Flexor hallucis longus

Peroneus brevis

Technique
Stand upright and take one big step backwards. Bend your back leg and push your heel towards the ground.

Muscles being stretched
Primary muscle: Soleus.
Secondary muscles: Tibialis posterior. Flexor hallucis longus. Flexor digitorum longus. Peroneus longus and brevis.

Sports that benefit from this stretch
Basketball. Netball. Boxing. Cycling. Hiking. Backpacking. Mountaineering. Orienteering. Ice hockey. Field hockey. Ice-skating. Roller-skating. Inline skating. Martial arts. Tennis. Badminton. Squash. Running. Track. Cross-country. American football (gridiron). Soccer. Rugby. Snow skiing. Water skiing. Surfing. Swimming. Walking. Race walking.

Sports injury where stretch may be useful
Calf strain. Achilles tendon strain. Achilles tendonitis. Medial tibial pain syndrome (shin splints). Posterior tibial tendonitis.

Common problems and more information for performing this stretch correctly
Make sure the toes of your back leg are facing forward. Letting your toes point to one side will cause this stretch to put uneven tension on the calf muscles. Over an extended period of time, this could lead to a muscle imbalance. Regulate the intensity of this stretch by lowering your body.

Complementary stretch
K05.

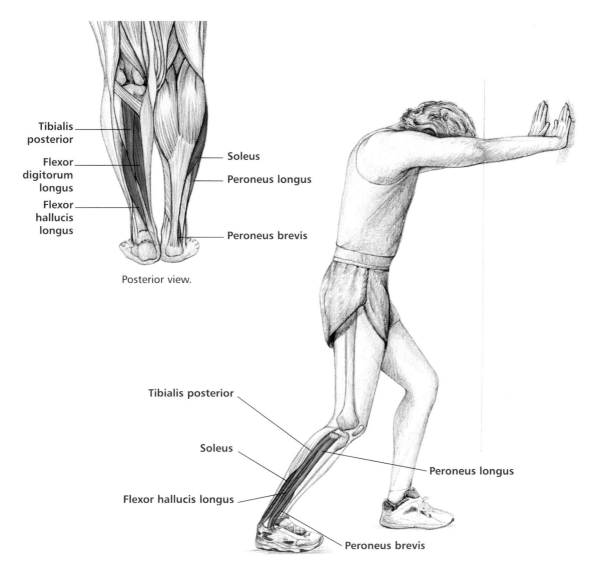

Posterior view.

Technique
Stand upright while leaning against a wall and place one foot behind the other. Make sure that both toes are facing forward and your heel is on the ground. Bend your back leg and lean towards the wall.

Muscles being stretched
Primary muscle: Soleus.
Secondary muscles: Tibialis posterior. Flexor hallucis longus. Flexor digitorum longus. Peroneus longus and brevis.

Sports that benefit from this stretch
Basketball. Netball. Boxing. Cycling. Hiking. Backpacking. Mountaineering. Orienteering. Ice hockey. Field hockey. Ice-skating. Roller-skating. Inline skating. Martial arts. Tennis. Badminton. Squash. Running. Track. Cross-country. American football (gridiron). Soccer. Rugby. Snow skiing. Water skiing. Surfing. Swimming. Walking. Race walking.

Sports injury where stretch may be useful
Calf strain. Achilles tendon strain. Achilles tendonitis. Medial tibial pain syndrome (shin splints). Posterior tibial tendonitis.

Common problems and more information for performing this stretch correctly
Make sure the toes of your back leg are facing forward. Letting your toes point to one side will cause this stretch to put uneven tension on the calf muscles. Over an extended period of time, this could lead to a muscle imbalance. Regulate the intensity of this stretch by lowering your body.

Complementary stretch
K02.

K05: SITTING BENT KNEE TOE PULL ACHILLES STRETCH

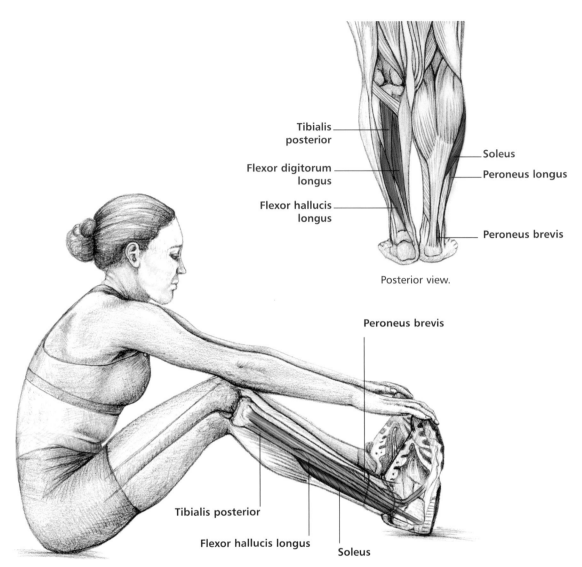

Tibialis posterior

Flexor digitorum longus

Flexor hallucis longus

Soleus

Peroneus longus

Peroneus brevis

Posterior view.

Peroneus brevis

Tibialis posterior

Flexor hallucis longus

Soleus

Technique
Sit with your legs out in front and bend both knees. Grab hold of your toes and pull them towards your knees.

Muscles being stretched
Primary muscle: Soleus.
Secondary muscles: Tibialis posterior. Flexor hallucis longus. Flexor digitorum longus. Peroneus longus and brevis.

Sports that benefit from this stretch
Basketball. Netball. Boxing. Cycling. Hiking. Backpacking. Mountaineering. Orienteering. Ice hockey. Field hockey. Ice-skating. Roller-skating. Inline skating. Martial arts. Tennis. Badminton. Squash. Running. Track. Cross-country. American football (gridiron). Soccer. Rugby. Snow skiing. Water skiing. Surfing. Swimming. Walking. Race walking.

Sports injury where stretch may be useful
Calf strain. Achilles tendon strain. Achilles tendonitis. Medial tibial pain syndrome (shin splints). Posterior tibial tendonitis.

Additional information for performing this stretch correctly
Regulate the intensity of this stretch by pushing your heels forward and pulling your toes back.

Complementary stretch
K01.

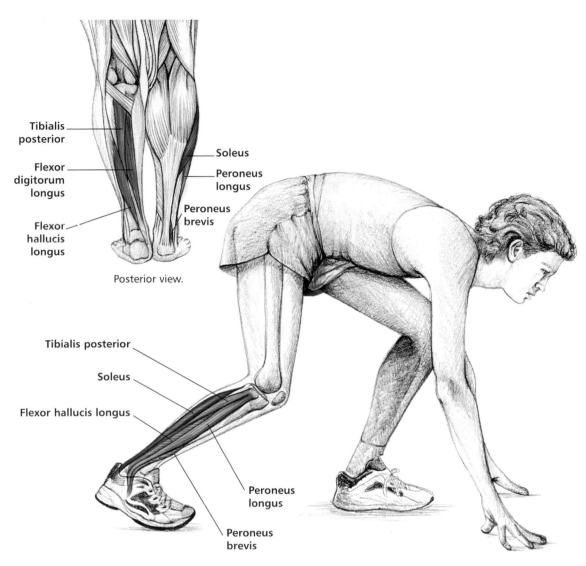

Posterior view.

Tibialis posterior
Flexor digitorum longus
Flexor hallucis longus
Soleus
Peroneus longus
Peroneus brevis

Tibialis posterior
Soleus
Flexor hallucis longus
Peroneus longus
Peroneus brevis

Technique

Stand upright and place one foot in front of the other. Bend both your front leg and your back leg and then push your back heel towards the ground. Lean forward and place your hands on the ground in front of you.

Muscles being stretched

Primary muscle: Soleus.
Secondary muscles: Tibialis posterior. Flexor hallucis longus. Flexor digitorum longus. Peroneus longus and brevis.

Sports that benefit from this stretch

Basketball. Netball. Boxing. Cycling. Hiking. Backpacking. Mountaineering. Orienteering. Ice hockey. Field hockey. Ice-skating. Roller-skating. Inline skating. Martial arts. Tennis. Badminton. Squash. Running. Track. Cross-country. American football (gridiron). Soccer. Rugby. Snow skiing. Water skiing. Surfing. Swimming. Walking. Race walking.

Sports injury where stretch may be useful

Calf strain. Achilles tendon strain. Achilles tendonitis. Medial tibial pain syndrome (shin splints). Posterior tibial tendonitis.

Common problems and more information for performing this stretch correctly

Make sure the toes of your back leg are facing forward. Letting your toes point to one side will cause this stretch to put uneven tension on the calf muscles. Over an extended period of time, this could lead to a muscle imbalance.

Complementary stretch

K04.

K07: KNEELING HEEL-DOWN ACHILLES STRETCH

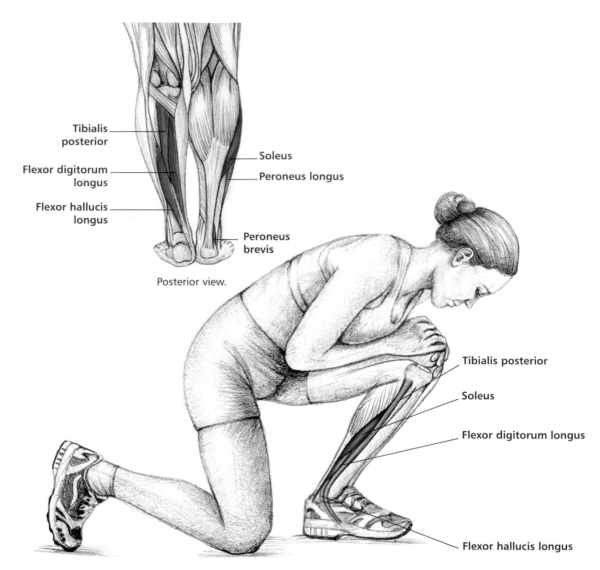

Tibialis posterior

Flexor digitorum longus

Flexor hallucis longus

Soleus

Peroneus longus

Peroneus brevis

Posterior view.

Tibialis posterior

Soleus

Flexor digitorum longus

Flexor hallucis longus

Technique
Kneel on one foot and place your body weight over your knee. Keep your heel on the ground and lean forward.

Muscles being stretched
Primary muscle: Soleus.
Secondary muscles: Tibialis posterior. Flexor hallucis longus. Flexor digitorum longus. Peroneus longus and brevis.

Sports that benefit from this stretch
Basketball. Netball. Boxing. Cycling. Hiking. Backpacking. Mountaineering. Orienteering. Ice hockey. Field hockey. Ice-skating. Roller-skating. Inline skating. Martial arts. Tennis. Badminton. Squash. Running. Track. Cross-country. American football (gridiron). Soccer. Rugby. Snow skiing. Water skiing. Surfing. Swimming. Walking. Race walking.

Sports injury where stretch may be useful
Calf strain. Achilles tendon strain. Achilles tendonitis. Medial tibial pain syndrome (shin splints). Posterior tibial tendonitis.

Common problems and more information for performing this stretch correctly
This stretch can put a lot of pressure on the Achilles tendon. Ease into this stretch by slowly leaning forward.

Complementary stretch
K01.

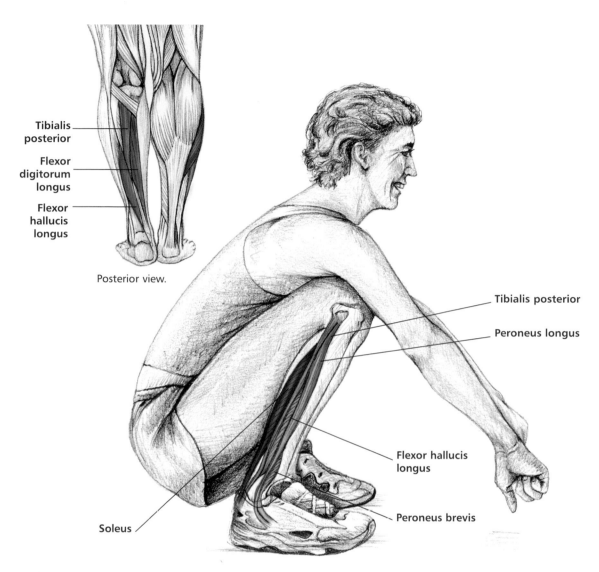

Tibialis posterior

Flexor digitorum longus

Flexor hallucis longus

Posterior view.

Tibialis posterior

Peroneus longus

Flexor hallucis longus

Peroneus brevis

Soleus

Technique
Stand with your feet at shoulder-width apart. Bend your legs and lower to a sitting position. Place your hands out in front for balance.

Muscles being stretched
Primary muscle: Soleus.
Secondary muscles: Tibialis posterior. Flexor hallucis longus. Flexor digitorum longus. Peroneus longus and brevis.

Sports that benefit from this stretch
Basketball. Netball. Boxing. Cycling. Hiking. Backpacking. Mountaineering. Orienteering. Ice hockey. Field hockey. Ice-skating. Roller-skating. Inline skating. Martial arts. Tennis. Badminton. Squash. Running. Track. Cross-country. American football (gridiron). Soccer. Rugby. Snow skiing. Water skiing. Surfing. Swimming. Walking. Race walking.

Sports injury where stretch may be useful
Calf strain. Achilles tendon strain. Achilles tendonitis. Medial tibial pain syndrome (shin splints). Posterior tibial tendonitis.

Additional information for performing this stretch correctly
If need be, hold onto something for balance and make sure your toes are facing forward.

Complementary stretch
K07.

14 Shins, Ankles, Feet, and Toes

The muscles of the shin originate at the top of the tibia, just below the knee joint, and extend down the front of the shin and over the ankle joint. The primary action of the shin muscles is to dorsiflex, extend, or invert the ankle joint.

The **extensor hallucis longus** and **extensor digitorum longus** are the main extensor muscles of the toes. The tendons of these muscles run over the front of the ankle, over the foot, and attach to the toes. These muscles dorsiflex the foot and work in opposition to the flexor muscles. When the calf muscles are tight, or the muscles are worked beyond their exertion level, inflammation of the tendon may occur.

Tibialis anterior originates from the lateral condyle of the tibia, and inserts into the medial and plantar surfaces of the medial cuneiform bone. Tibialis anterior is responsible for dorsiflexing and inverting the foot and is used frequently during running to *toe up* with each step. Pain in the front of the shin occurs when the muscle and tendon become inflamed and irritated through overuse or improper form.

One structure worth noting is a tough fibrous tissue, **plantar fascia**, also called *plantar aponeurosis*, which connects the heel to the toes. Repetitive ankle movement, especially when restricted by tight calves, can irritate this tissue at the insertion on the heel. Specific stretches later in this chapter help to alleviate this problem.

The feet and ankles are comprised of a multitude of small muscles that control the foot. The muscles around the feet and ankles, along with the structure of the joints, allow for a large range of movement of the feet and ankles, including: plantar flexion, dorsiflexion, inversion, eversion, and rotation.

There are four layers of muscle in the sole of the foot. The first layer is the most inferior (that is, the most superficial and closest to the ground in standing), comprising **abductor hallucis, flexor digitorum brevis**, and **abductor digiti minimi.** Abductor digiti minimi forms the lateral margin of the sole of the foot. The second layer contains the **lumbricales** and **quadratus plantae,** plus the tendons of flexor hallucis longus and flexor digitorum longus. The third layer contains **flexor hallucis brevis**, **adductor hallucis**, and **flexor digiti minimi brevis**. The fourth layer is the deepest (most superior) layer of muscles of the sole of the foot. It consists of the four muscles of the dorsal interossei, the three muscles of the plantar interossei, and the tendons of tibialis posterior and peroneus longus. On the dorsum of the foot lies extensor digitorum brevis.

Sports that benefit from these shin, ankles, and feet stretches include: basketball and netball; boxing; cycling; hiking, backpacking, mountaineering, and orienteering; ice hockey and field hockey; ice-skating, roller-skating, and inline skating; martial arts; racquet sports like tennis, badminton, and squash; running, track, and cross-country; running sports like soccer, American football (gridiron), and rugby; snow skiing and water skiing; surfing; swimming; walking and race walking.

L01: FOOT-BEHIND SHIN STRETCH

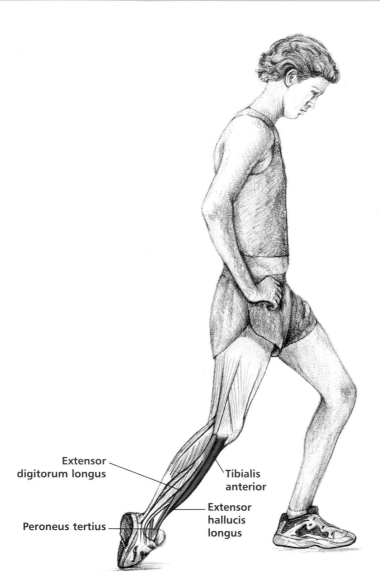

Extensor digitorum longus

Tibialis anterior

Extensor hallucis longus

Peroneus tertius

Technique
Stand upright and place the top of your toes on the ground behind you. Push your ankle to the ground.

Muscles being stretched
Primary muscle: Tibialis anterior.
Secondary muscles: Extensor hallucis longus. Extensor digitorum longus. Peroneus tertius.

Sports that benefit from this stretch
Basketball. Netball. Boxing. Hiking. Backpacking. Mountaineering. Orienteering. Martial arts. Tennis. Badminton. Squash. Running. Track. Cross-country. American football (gridiron). Soccer. Rugby. Walking. Race walking.

Sports injury where stretch may be useful
Anterior compartment syndrome. Medial tibial pain syndrome (shin splints). Ankle sprain. Peroneal tendon subluxation. Peroneal tendonitis.

Additional information for performing this stretch correctly
Regulate the intensity of this stretch by lowering your body and pushing your ankle to the ground. If need be, hold onto something for balance.

Complementary stretch
L02.

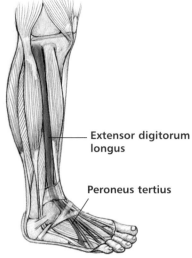

Extensor digitorum longus

Peroneus tertius

Right leg, lateral view.

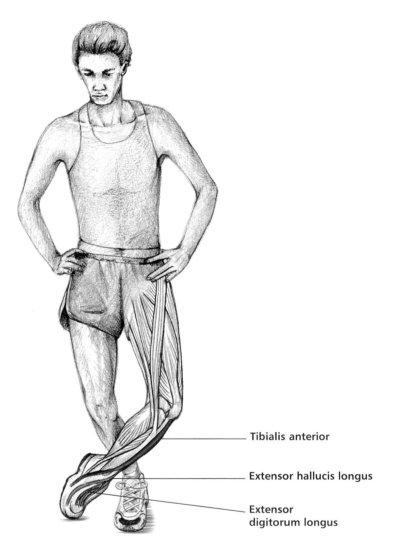

Tibialis anterior

Extensor hallucis longus

Extensor digitorum longus

Technique
Stand upright and place the top of your toes on the ground in front of your other foot. Slowly bend your other leg to force your ankle to the ground.

Muscles being stretched
Primary muscle: Tibialis anterior.
Secondary muscles: Extensor hallucis longus. Extensor digitorum longus. Peroneus tertius.

Sports that benefit from this stretch
Basketball. Netball. Boxing. Hiking. Backpacking. Mountaineering. Orienteering. Martial arts. Tennis. Badminton. Squash. Running. Track. Cross-country. American football (gridiron). Soccer. Rugby. Walking. Race walking.

Sports injury where stretch may be useful
Anterior compartment syndrome. Medial tibial pain syndrome (shin splints). Ankle sprain. Peroneal tendon subluxation. Peroneal tendonitis.

Additional information for performing this stretch correctly
Regulate the intensity of this stretch by lowering your body.

Complementary stretch
L04.

L03: RAISED FOOT SHIN STRETCH

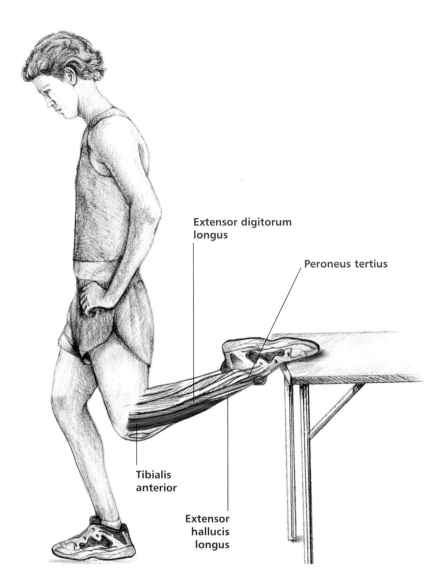

Extensor digitorum longus

Peroneus tertius

Tibialis anterior

Extensor hallucis longus

Technique
Stand upright and place the top of your toes on a raised object behind you. Push your ankle downwards.

Muscles being stretched
Primary muscle: Tibialis anterior.
Secondary muscles: Extensor hallucis longus.
Extensor digitorum longus. Peroneus tertius.

Sports that benefit from this stretch
Basketball. Netball. Boxing. Hiking. Backpacking.
Mountaineering. Orienteering. Martial arts.
Tennis. Badminton. Squash. Running. Track.
Cross-country. American football (gridiron).
Soccer. Rugby. Walking. Race walking.

Sports injury where stretch may be useful
Anterior compartment syndrome. Medial tibial pain syndrome (shin splints). Ankle sprain.
Peroneal tendon subluxation. Peroneal tendonitis.

Additional information for performing this stretch correctly
If need be, hold onto something for balance.

Complementary stretch
L01.

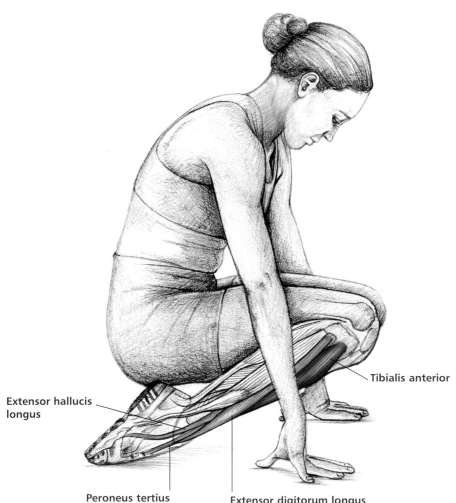

Tibialis anterior

Extensor hallucis longus

Peroneus tertius

Extensor digitorum longus

Technique
Sit with your knees and feet flat on the ground. Sit back on your ankles and keep your heels and knees together. Place your hands next to your knees and slowly lean backwards. Slowly raise your knees off the ground.

Muscles being stretched
Primary muscle: Tibialis anterior.
Secondary muscles: Extensor hallucis longus. Extensor digitorum longus. Peroneus tertius.

Sports that benefit from this stretch
Basketball. Netball. Boxing. Hiking. Backpacking. Mountaineering. Orienteering. Martial arts. Tennis. Badminton. Squash. Running. Track. Cross-country. American football (gridiron). Soccer. Rugby. Walking. Race walking.

Sports injury where stretch may be useful
Anterior compartment syndrome. Medial tibial pain syndrome (shin splints). Ankle sprain. Peroneal tendon subluxation. Peroneal tendonitis.

Common problems and more information for performing this stretch correctly
This stretch can put a lot of pressure on your knees and ankles. Do not attempt this stretch if you suffer from knee or ankle pain.

Complementary stretch
L03.

L05: SQUATTING TOE STRETCH

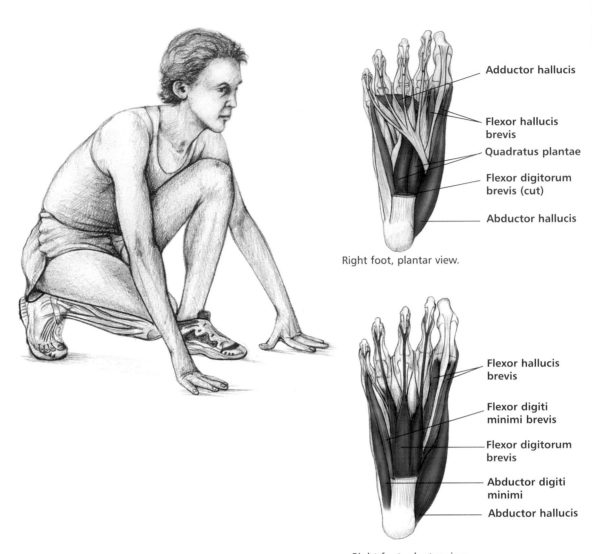

Right foot, plantar view.

Adductor hallucis
Flexor hallucis brevis
Quadratus plantae
Flexor digitorum brevis (cut)
Abductor hallucis

Flexor hallucis brevis
Flexor digiti minimi brevis
Flexor digitorum brevis
Abductor digiti minimi
Abductor hallucis

Right foot, plantar view.

Technique
Kneel on one foot with your hands on the ground. Place your body weight over your knee and slowly move your knee forward. Keep your toes on the ground and arch your foot.

Muscles being stretched
Primary muscles: Flexor digitorum brevis. Abductor hallucis. Abductor digiti minimi. Quadratus plantae.
Secondary muscles: Flexor hallucis brevis. Adductor hallucis. Flexor digiti minimi brevis.

Sports that benefit from this stretch
Basketball. Netball. Boxing. Cycling. Hiking. Backpacking. Mountaineering. Orienteering. Martial arts. Tennis. Badminton. Squash. Running. Track. Cross-country. American football (gridiron). Soccer. Rugby. Surfing. Walking. Race walking.

Sports injury where stretch may be useful
Posterior tibial tendonitis. Peroneal tendon subluxation. Peroneal tendonitis. Flexor tendonitis. Sesamoiditis. Plantar fasciitis.

Common problems and additional information for performing this stretch correctly
The muscles and tendons underneath the foot can be very tight; do not apply too much force too quickly when doing this stretch.

Complementary stretch
K07.

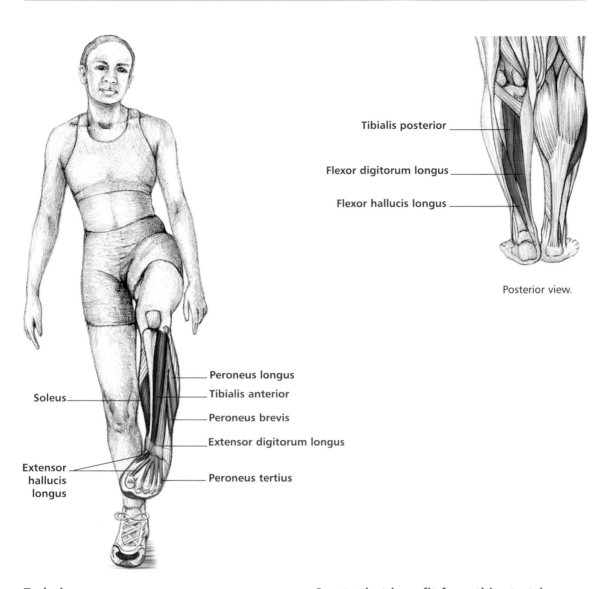

Tibialis posterior

Flexor digitorum longus

Flexor hallucis longus

Posterior view.

Peroneus longus

Tibialis anterior

Soleus

Peroneus brevis

Extensor digitorum longus

Extensor
hallucis
longus

Peroneus tertius

Technique
Raise one foot off the ground and slowly rotate your foot and ankle in all directions.

Muscles being stretched
Primary muscles: Soleus. Tibialis anterior. Secondary muscles: Extensor hallucis longus. Extensor digitorum longus. Peroneus longus, brevis, and tertius. Tibialis posterior. Flexor hallucis longus. Flexor digitorum longus.

Sports that benefit from this stretch
Basketball. Netball. Boxing. Hiking. Backpacking. Mountaineering. Orienteering. Martial arts. Tennis. Badminton. Squash. Running. Track. Cross-country. American football (gridiron). Soccer. Rugby. Walking. Race walking.

Sports that benefit from this stretch
Anterior compartment syndrome. Medial tibial pain syndrome (shin splints). Ankle sprain. Posterior tibial tendonitis. Peroneal tendon subluxation. Peroneal tendonitis.

Additional information for performing this stretch correctly
If need be, hold onto something for balance.

Complementary stretches
L02, K02.

Resources

Alter, M.J.: 2004. *Science of Flexibility.* Human Kinetics. IL, USA.

Anderson, R. A.: 2010. *Stretching.* Shelter Publications. CA, USA.

Armiger, P.: 2010. *Stretching for Functional Flexibility.* Lippincott, Williams & Wilkins. MD, USA.

Bahr, R. & Maehlum, S.: 2004. *Clinical Guide to Sports Injuries.* Human Kinetics. IL, USA.

Beachle, T. & Earle, R.: 2008. *Essentials of Strength Training and Conditioning.* Human Kinetics. IL, USA.

Biel, A.: 2010. *Trail Guide to the Body.* Books of Discovery. CO, USA.

Chek, P.: 2009. *An Integrated Approach to Stretching.* C.H.E.K. Institute. CA, USA.

Delavier, F.: 2010. *Strength Training Anatomy.* Human Kinetics. IL, USA.

Goldspink, G.: 1968. Sarcomere length during post-natal growth and mammalian muscle fibers. *Journal of Cell Science,* 3(4): 539–548.

Gummerson, T.: 1990. *Mobility Training for the Martial Arts.* A & C Black. London, UK.

Jarmey, C.: 2008. *The Concise Book of Muscles.* Lotus Publishing. Chichester, UK.

Jarmey, C.: 2006. *The Concise Book of the Moving Body.* Lotus Publishing. Chichester, UK.

Kurz, T.: 2003. *Stretching Scientifically.* Stadion Publishing Company. VT, USA.

Martini, F., Timmons, M. & Tallitsch, R.: 2009. *Human Anatomy.* Pearson Benjamin Cummings. CA, USA.

Mattes, A.: 2000. *Active Isolated Stretching: The Mattes Method.* Self Published. FL, USA.

McAtee, R. & Charland, J.: 2007. *Facilitated Stretching.* Human Kinetics. IL, USA.

Norris, C.M.: 1998. *Sports Injuries: Diagnosis and Management.* Butterworth-Heinemann. Oxford, UK.

Tortora, G.J. & Derrickson, B.: 2009. *Principles of Anatomy and Physiology.* John Wiley & Sons, Inc. NJ, USA.

Walker, B.: 2007. *The Stretching Handbook.* The Stretching Institute. NY, USA.

Walker, B.: 2007. *The Anatomy of Sports Injuries.* Lotus Publishing. Chichester, UK.

Weldon, S.M.: 2003. The efficacy of stretching for prevention of exercise-related injury: a systematic review of the literature. *Manual Therapy,* 8(3): 141.

Wharton, J & P.: 1996. *The Whartons' Stretch Book.* Three Rivers Press. NY, USA.

Williams, P.E. & Goldspink, G.: 1971. Longitudinal growth of striated muscle fibers. *Journal of Cell Science,* 9(3): 751–767.

Wilmore, J.H. & Costill, D.L.: 1994. *Physiology of Sport and Exercise.* Human Kinetics. IL, USA.

Ylinen, J.: 2008. *Stretching Therapy.* Elsevier. PA, USA.

Top Five Stretches for Each Sports Injury

The stretches below are a short list of suggested stretches to help with a number of common sports injuries. The following stretches are beneficial for the prevention and long-term rehabilitation of the injuries listed below; however, they are not to be used in the initial stages of injury rehabilitation. Stretching during this early stage of the rehabilitation process will only cause more damage to the injured tissues. Avoid all stretching during the first seventy-two hours after any soft tissue injury, and remember to follow *The Rules for Safe Stretching* in Chapter 2.

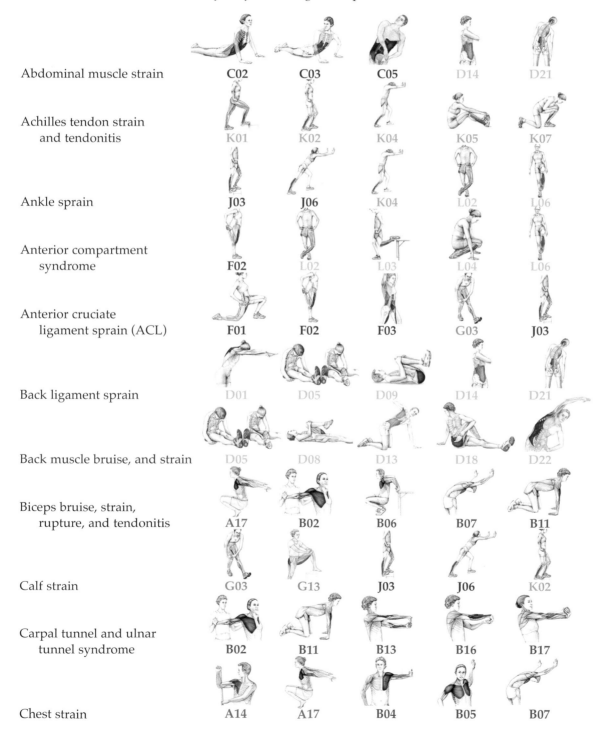

Injury					
Abdominal muscle strain	C02	C03	C05	D14	D21
Achilles tendon strain and tendonitis	K01	K02	K04	K05	K07
Ankle sprain	J03	J06	K04	L02	L06
Anterior compartment syndrome	F02	L02	L03	L04	L06
Anterior cruciate ligament sprain (ACL)	F01	F02	F03	G03	J03
Back ligament sprain	D01	D05	D09	D14	D21
Back muscle bruise, and strain	D05	D08	D13	D18	D22
Biceps bruise, strain, rupture, and tendonitis	A17	B02	B06	B07	B11
Calf strain	G03	G13	J03	J06	K02
Carpal tunnel and ulnar tunnel syndrome	B02	B11	B13	B16	B17
Chest strain	A14	A17	B04	B05	B07

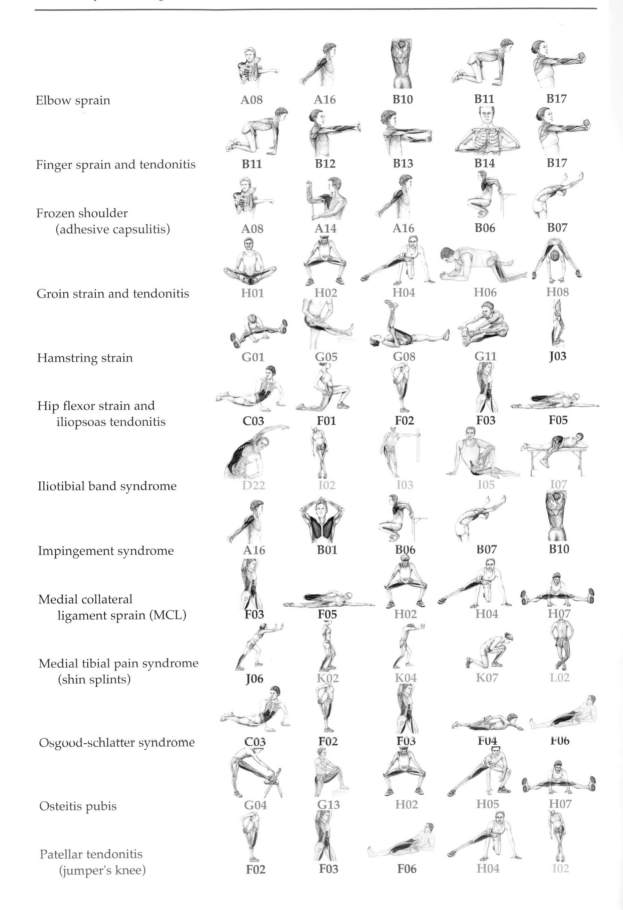

Elbow sprain	A08	A16	B10	B11	B17
Finger sprain and tendonitis	B11	B12	B13	B14	B17
Frozen shoulder (adhesive capsulitis)	A08	A14	A16	B06	B07
Groin strain and tendonitis	H01	H02	H04	H06	H08
Hamstring strain	G01	G05	G08	G11	J03
Hip flexor strain and iliopsoas tendonitis	C03	F01	F02	F03	F05
Iliotibial band syndrome	D22	I02	I03	I05	I07
Impingement syndrome	A16	B01	B06	B07	B10
Medial collateral ligament sprain (MCL)	F03	F05	H02	H04	H07
Medial tibial pain syndrome (shin splints)	J06	K02	K04	K07	L02
Osgood-schlatter syndrome	C03	F02	F03	F04	F06
Osteitis pubis	G04	G13	H02	H05	H07
Patellar tendonitis (jumper's knee)	F02	F03	F06	H04	I02

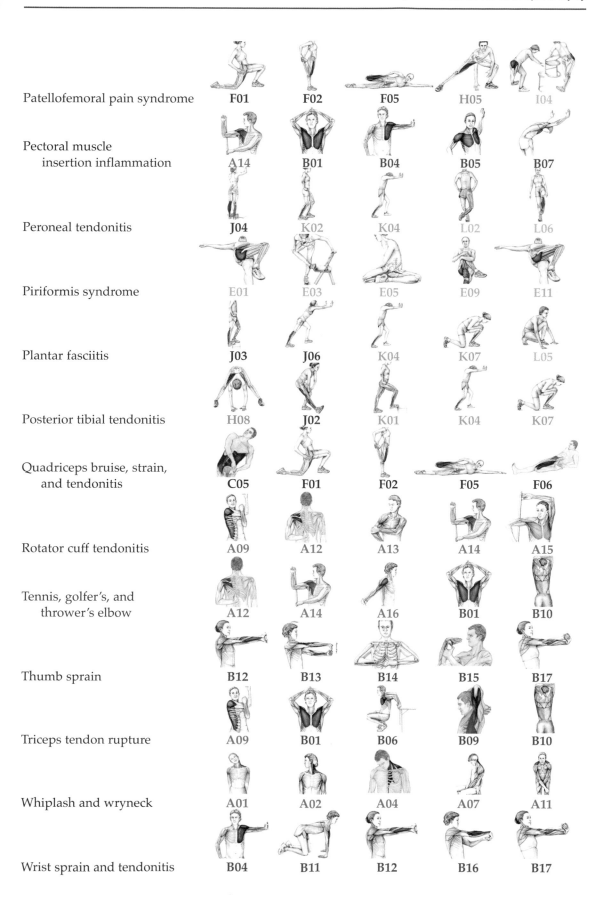

Patellofemoral pain syndrome	F01	F02	F05	H05	I04
Pectoral muscle insertion inflammation	A14	B01	B04	B05	B07
Peroneal tendonitis	J04	K02	K04	L02	L06
Piriformis syndrome	E01	E03	E05	E09	E11
Plantar fasciitis	J03	J06	K04	K07	L05
Posterior tibial tendonitis	H08	J02	K01	K04	K07
Quadriceps bruise, strain, and tendonitis	C05	F01	F02	F05	F06
Rotator cuff tendonitis	A09	A12	A13	A14	A15
Tennis, golfer's, and thrower's elbow	A12	A14	A16	B01	B10
Thumb sprain	B12	B13	B14	B15	B17
Triceps tendon rupture	A09	B01	B06	B09	B10
Whiplash and wryneck	A01	A02	A04	A07	A11
Wrist sprain and tendonitis	B04	B11	B12	B16	B17

Top Five Stretches for Each Sport

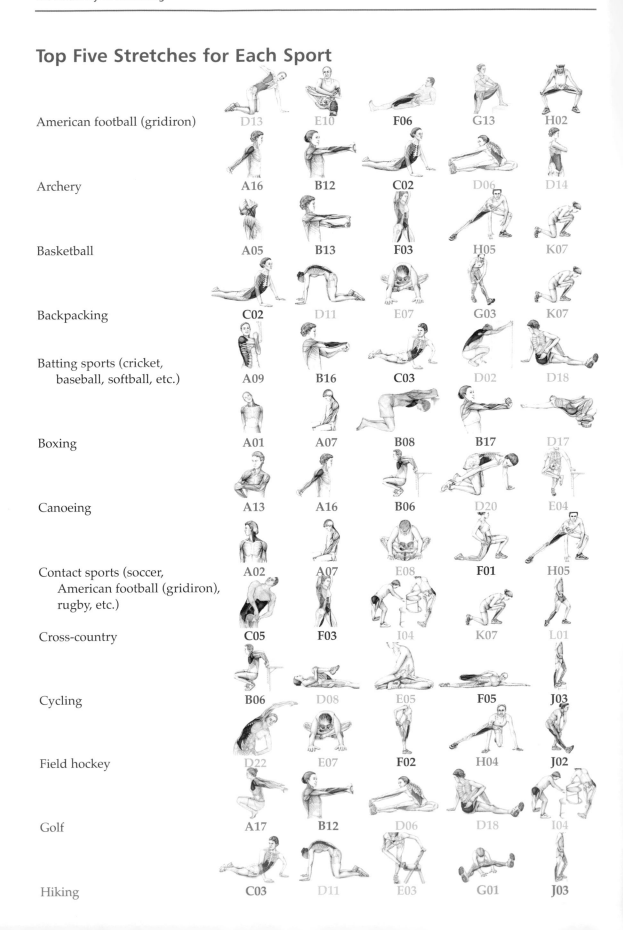

Sport					
American football (gridiron)	D13	E10	**F06**	G13	H02
Archery	A16	**B12**	**C02**	D06	D14
Basketball	A05	**B13**	**F03**	H05	K07
Backpacking	**C02**	D11	E07	G03	K07
Batting sports (cricket, baseball, softball, etc.)	A09	**B16**	**C03**	D02	D18
Boxing	A01	A07	**B08**	**B17**	D17
Canoeing	A13	A16	**B06**	D20	E04
Contact sports (soccer, American football (gridiron), rugby, etc.)	A02	A07	E08	**F01**	H05
Cross-country	**C05**	**F03**	I04	K07	L01
Cycling	**B06**	D08	E05	**F05**	**J03**
Field hockey	D22	E07	**F02**	H04	**J02**
Golf	A17	**B12**	D06	D18	I04
Hiking	**C03**	D11	E03	G01	J03

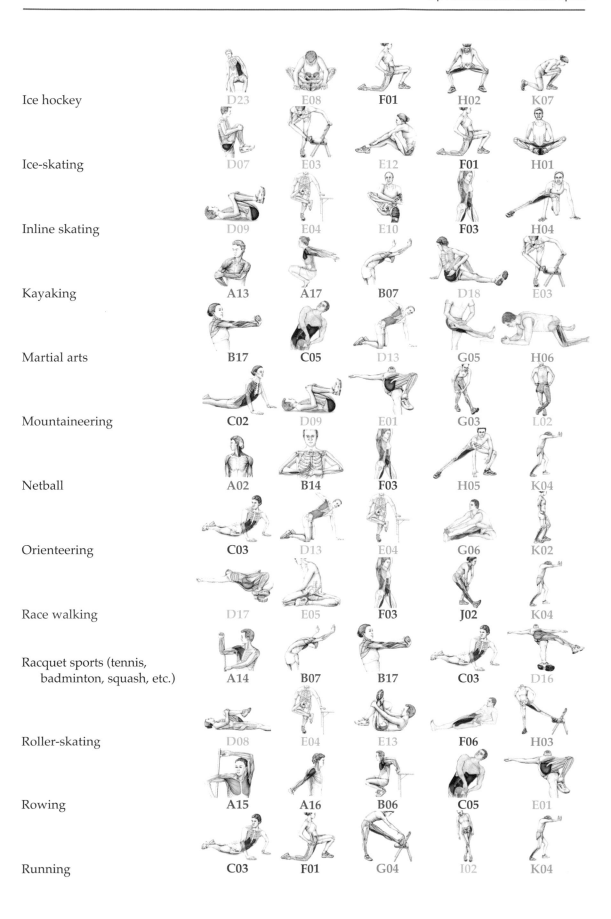

Ice hockey	D23	E08	**F01**	H02	K07
Ice-skating	D07	E03	E12	**F01**	H01
Inline skating	D09	E04	E10	**F03**	H04
Kayaking	**A13**	**A17**	**B07**	D18	E03
Martial arts	**B17**	**C05**	D13	**G05**	**H06**
Mountaineering	**C02**	D09	E01	**G03**	L02
Netball	**A02**	**B14**	**F03**	H05	K04
Orienteering	**C03**	D13	E04	**G06**	K02
Race walking	D17	E05	**F03**	**J02**	K04
Racquet sports (tennis, badminton, squash, etc.)	**A14**	**B07**	**B17**	**C03**	D16
Roller-skating	D08	E04	E13	**F06**	H03
Rowing	**A15**	**A16**	**B06**	**C05**	E01
Running	**C03**	**F01**	**G04**	I02	K04

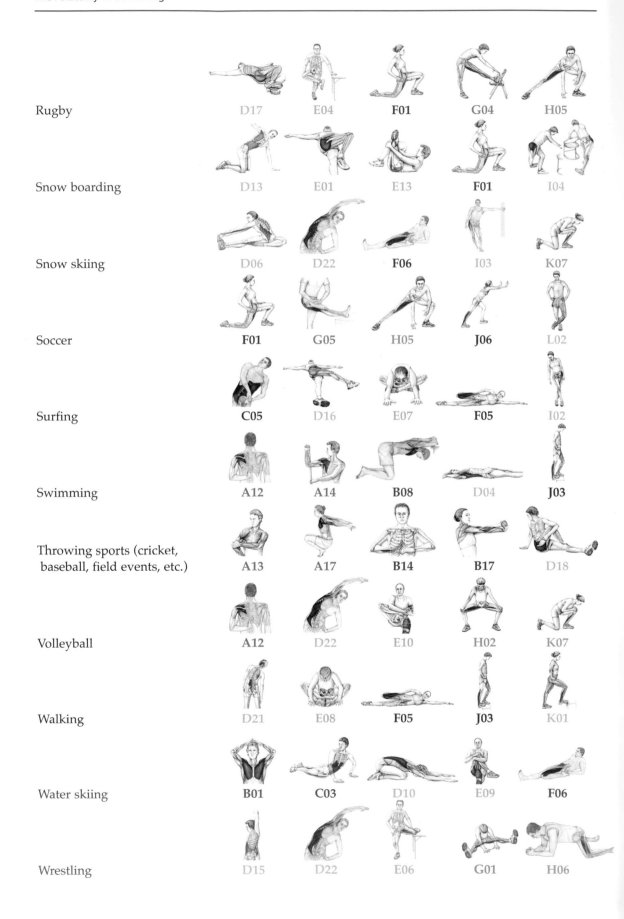

Rugby	D17	E04	**F01**	G04	H05
Snow boarding	D13	E01	E13	**F01**	I04
Snow skiing	D06	D22	**F06**	I03	K07
Soccer	**F01**	G05	H05	**J06**	L02
Surfing	**C05**	D16	E07	**F05**	I02
Swimming	**A12**	**A14**	**B08**	D04	**J03**
Throwing sports (cricket, baseball, field events, etc.)	**A13**	**A17**	**B14**	**B17**	D18
Volleyball	**A12**	D22	E10	**H02**	K07
Walking	D21	E08	**F05**	**J03**	K01
Water skiing	**B01**	**C03**	D10	E09	**F06**
Wrestling	D15	D22	E06	**G01**	**H06**

Glossary

Achilles tendonitis Inflammation of the Achilles tendon.
Adhesive capsulitis Adhesive inflammation between the joint capsule and the peripheral articular cartilage of the shoulder. Causes pain, stiffness, and limitation of movement. Also known as frozen shoulder.
Ankylosing spondylitis Form of degenerative joint disease that affects the spine. Systemic illness, producing pain and stiffness as a result of inflammation of the sacroiliac, intervertebral, and costovertebral joints.
Anterior tibial compartment syndrome Rapid swelling, increased tension, and pain of the anterior tibial compartment of the leg. Usually a history of excessive exertion.
Arthropathy Any joint disease.
Articular dysfunction Disturbance, impairment, or abnormality of a joint.
Avulsion fracture Indirect fracture caused by compressive forces from direct trauma or excessive tensile forces.

Bursa Fibrous sac membrane containing synovial fluid, typically found between tendons and bones. It acts to reduce friction during movement.
Bursitis Inflammation of the bursa, e.g., subdeltoid bursa.

Calcific tendonitis Inflammation and calcification of the subacromial or subdeltoid bursa. This results in pain, and limitation of movement of the shoulder.
Capsulitis Inflammation of a capsule, e.g., joint.
Carpal tunnel syndrome Compression of the median nerve as it passes through the carpal tunnel, leading to pain and tingling in the hand.
Cervical nerve stretch syndrome Condition caused by irritation or compression of the cervical nerve roots by a protruding disc.
Coccydynia Pain in the coccyx and neighbouring region. Also known as coccygodynia.
Compartment syndrome Condition in which increased intramuscular pressure impedes blood flow and function of tissues within that compartment.

Discogenic pain Pain caused by derangement of an intervertebral disc.
Dislocation The displacement of any part, especially of a bone.

Epicondylitis Inflammation and microrupturing of the soft tissues on the epicondyles of the distal humerus.

Fasciitis Inflammation of the fascia surrounding portions of a muscle.
Frozen shoulder syndrome see adhesive capsulitis.

Golfer's elbow Inflammation of the medial epicondyle of the humerus caused by activities (e.g., golf) that involve gripping and twisting, especially when there is a forceful grip.

Heel spur Bony spur from the calcaneum.

Iliotibial band syndrome Pain/inflammation of the iliotibial band (ITB), a non-elastic collagen cord stretching from the pelvis to below the knee. There are various biomechanical causes.
Impingement syndrome Chronic condition caused by a repetitive overhead activity that damages the glenoid labrum, long head of the biceps brachii, and subacromial bursa.
Inflammation A localized protective response caused by injury to tissues. Characterized by pain, heat, redness, swelling, and loss of function.

Lordosis Excessive convex curve in the lumbar region of the spine.

Medial tibial pain syndrome Rapid swelling, increased tension, and pain of the medial tibial compartment of the leg. Usually a history of excessive exertion. Also known as shin splints.

Neuritis Inflammation of a nerve, with pain and tenderness.

Osteitis Inflammation of a bone, causing enlargement of the bone, tenderness, and a dull, aching pain.
Osteitis pubis A symptom-producing inflammatory condition of the pubic bones in the region of the symphysis. May be caused by a variety of conditions including degenerative changes.
Osteoarthritis Non-inflammatory degenerative joint disease, characterized by degeneration of the articular cartilage, hypertrophy of bone at the margins, and changes in the synovial membrane. Seen particularly in older persons.

Patellofemoral pain syndrome Excessive pain pertaining to the patella and femur.
Piriformis syndrome Condition resulting from the muscle being inflamed, shortened, or in spasm, causing impingement on the sciatic nerve. Causes pain and tingling in the posterior thigh and buttock. Occurs more frequently in women than men (ratio 6:1).

Repetitive strain injury (RSI) Refers to any overuse condition, such as strain, or tendonitis in any part of the body.
Rheumatoid arthritis Autoimmune disease, in which the immune system attacks the body's own tissues. Causes inflammation of many parts of the body.
Rotator cuff Helps hold the head of the humerus in contact with the glenoid cavity (fossa, socket) of the scapula during movements of the shoulder, thus helping to prevent dislocation of the joint. Comprises of: supraspinatus, infraspinatus, teres minor, and subscapularis.
Rupture Forcible tearing or disruption of tissue.

Sacroiliitis Inflammation (arthritis) in the sacroiliac joint.
Scapulocostal syndrome Pain in the superior or posterior aspect of the shoulder girdle, as a result of long-standing alteration of the relationship of the scapula and the posterior thoracic wall.
Scoliosis Lateral rotational spinal curvature.
Sesamoid bone Small nodular bones embedded in a tendon or joint.
Sesamoiditis Inflammation of the sesamoid bones and surrounding structures.
Shin splints see medial tibial pain syndrome/anterior tibial compartment syndrome.
Snapping hip syndrome Possibly caused by tight ligaments and tendons passing over bony prominences. Internal snapping mainly caused by the suction phenomenon, occurring during exercises such as sit-ups. External snapping usually as a result of the gluteus maximus clicking over the greater trochanter. Common in dancers and young athletes. Also known as clicking hip syndrome.
Sprain Joint injury in which some of the fibres of a supporting ligament are ruptured.
Strain An overstretching or overexertion of some part of the musculature.
Subluxation An incomplete or partial dislocation.

Tendonitis Inflammation of a tendon. Also known as tendinitis.
Tennis elbow Tendonitis of the muscles of the back of the forearm at their insertion. Caused by excessive hammering or sawing type movements, or a tense, awkward grip on a tennis racquet.
Tenosynovitis Inflammation of a tendon sheath.
Thrower's elbow Repetitive stress to the medial collateral ligament.
Torticollis Contracted state of the cervical muscles, producing twisting of the neck.
Trochanteric bursitis Trochanteric bursa lies between gluteus maximus and the posterolateral surface of the greater trochanter. Bursitis may occur if flexibility of the iliotibial band (ITB) is reduced.

Ulnar tunnel syndrome The ulnar nerve runs down the inside of the forearm to the heel of the hand. Excessive pressure on this nerve can cause numbness and tingling that is confined to the little finger and the outside of the ring finger. Usually not caused by repetitive motions.

Whiplash Nonspecific term applied to injury to the spine and spinal cord at C4/C5, occurring as the result of rapid acceleration/deceleration of the body.
Wry neck see torticollis.